When Someone
You Know
Is Living in a
Dementia Care
Community

A 36-Hour Day Book

When Someone You Know Is Living in a Dementia Care Community

WORDS TO SAY *and* THINGS TO DO

Rachael Wonderlin

Johns Hopkins University Press
Baltimore

This book is not meant to substitute for medical, legal, or other professional care of people with dementia, and treatment should not be based solely on its contents. Instead, treatment must be developed in a dialogue between the individual and his or her physician. This book has been written to help with that dialogue.

Johns Hopkins University Press
2715 North Charles Street
Baltimore, Maryland 21218-4363
www.press.jhu.edu

Library of Congress Cataloging-in-Publication Data

Names: Wonderlin, Rachael, 1989–, author.
Title: When someone you know is living in a dementia care community /
    Rachael Wonderlin.
Description: Baltimore : Johns Hopkins University Press, 2016. |
    Includes bibliographical references and index.
Identifiers: LCCN 2015050731| ISBN 9781421420646 (hardcover : alk. paper) |
    ISBN 1421420643 (hardcover : alk. paper) | ISBN 9781421420653
    (pbk. : alk. paper) | ISBN 1421420651 (pbk. : alk. paper) |
    ISBN 9781421420660 (electronic) | ISBN 142142066X (electronic)
Subjects: LCSH: Dementia—Patients—Care. | Older people—Care. |
    Long-term care facilities. | Popular works.
Classification: LCC RC521.W63 2016 | DDC 616.8/3—dc23
LC record available at http://lccn.loc.gov/2015050731

A catalog record for this book is available from the British Library.

Special discounts are available for bulk purchases of this book. For more information, please contact Special Sales at 410-516-6936 or specialsales@press.jhu.edu.

Johns Hopkins University Press uses environmentally friendly book materials, including recycled text paper that is composed of at least 30 percent post-consumer waste, whenever possible.

This book is for my grandparents, Paul, Patti, Eugene, and Charlotte, who showed me that aging can be graceful, happy, and full of love and wisdom. This is for everyone who encouraged me along the way—especially my family, Rob, my professors from the University of Mary Washington Psychology Department and UNC Greensboro, and a lot of great friends.

And for Dot, who showed me that dementia can never rob you of what makes you beautiful.

Contents

PART IV

RELATIONSHIPS AND DEMENTIA

PART V

CHALLENGES AND CHANGES IN ADVANCED DEMENTIA CARE

Preface

Dementia can be a lonely diagnosis, especially for the caregiver. Spouses, partners, adult children, siblings, close friends—whoever the caregivers are, their challenges are many. And their questions are many, too.

- Is long-term care right for my family member or friend with dementia?
- What happens after I drop my parent, partner, sibling, child, or friend off at a long-term-care community?
- What should I do to prepare for move-in day?
- How can I make my visits go more smoothly?
- What happens if my loved one has a romantic relationship with another resident?

Even if you are the person who has made the difficult decision to bring a family member or friend to a long-term-care community, you may feel like you don't have all the answers you need or anywhere to turn to get them. Most of the information found online and in other books focuses on in-home care. Although this information is useful, people looking into dementia care communities need information specifically about community dementia care.

Maybe you have yet to choose a long-term-care community for your loved one, but you can see that the choice is on the horizon. Maybe in-home care has become too challenging or too exhausting. Perhaps you have been the sole caregiver for years, but you know that now you must focus on yourself.

Maybe you aren't thinking about these decisions for someone you know but instead work in a long-term-care community and want to gain even more insight into the people you help care for. Maybe you are a student who is curious to learn more about dementia care. In any case, I hope this book provides you with many of the answers you seek. My goal is to improve your relationship with the cognitively impaired individual or individuals in your life while helping you choose the best long-term dementia care community possible.

When discussing long-term care in this book, I will use the term "communities" to describe places where people who have dementia live. Other terms, such as "homes" or "facilities," are often used, but I find the word "communities" to be friendlier. Despite the many types of long-term care—in-home care, assisted-living communities, independent-living communities, continuing-care retirement communities, and skilled-nursing facilities—this book will focus on dementia care within a community. I will not use the phrase "memory-care community" because not all residents in a dementia care community have a memory problem. In this book all these communities will be called "dementia care communities."

I tell many stories about families and residents, but their names and the details of their lives have been changed to protect their identities.

Before going further, I want to pause to share my list of things I would want if I had dementia. This was originally posted on my friend Bob DeMarco's popular blog, Alzheimer's Reading Room. The list captures the essence of the book you are about to read. It has helped many caregivers preserve the wishes of the *person* in the person who has dementia.

16 Things I Would Want If I Got Dementia

1. If I get dementia, I want my friends and family to embrace my reality. If I think my spouse is still alive, or if I think we're visiting my parents for dinner, let me believe those things. I'll be much happier for it.
2. If I get dementia, I don't want to be treated like a child. Talk to me like the adult that I am.
3. If I get dementia, I still want to enjoy the things that I've always enjoyed. Help me find a way to exercise, read, and visit with friends.

4. If I get dementia, ask me to tell you a story from my past.

5. If I get dementia, and I become agitated, take the time to figure out what is bothering me.

6. If I get dementia, treat me the way that you would want to be treated.

7. If I get dementia, make sure that there are plenty of snacks for me in the house. Even now if I don't eat I get angry, and if I have dementia, I may have trouble explaining what I need.

8. If I get dementia, don't talk about me as if I'm not in the room.

9. If I get dementia, don't feel guilty if you cannot care for me 24 hours a day, 7 days a week. It's not your fault, and you've done your best. Find someone who can help you, or choose a great new place for me to live.

10. If I get dementia, and I live in a dementia care community, please visit me often.

11. If I get dementia, don't act frustrated if I mix up names, events, or places. Take a deep breath. It's not my fault.

12. If I get dementia, make sure I always have my favorite music playing within earshot.

13. If I get dementia, and I like to pick up items and carry them around, help me return those items to their original places.

14. If I get dementia, don't exclude me from parties and family gatherings.

15. If I get dementia, know that I still like receiving hugs or handshakes.

16. If I get dementia, remember that I am still the person you know and love.

PART I

BASICS OF DEMENTIA CARE, AND LIFE IN A DEMENTIA CARE COMMUNITY

1

What Is Long-Term Care?

Long-term care is a group of services and communities that cater to aging adults. The many types of long-term care include

in-home care, plus
assisted-living,
personal-care,
independent-living,
skilled-nursing,
adult day-care, and
dementia care communities.

In some cases, dementia care communities, or units, are part of a larger community. For example, some assisted-living or personal-care communities have their own dementia care wing.

Dementia care communities differ from other types of communities in a few key ways. Unlike assisted-living facilities (ALFs) and skilled-nursing facilities (SNFs, often called "nursing homes"), dementia care communities cater to those with dementia. Residents of ALFs do not necessarily have dementia, and they are typically more physically and cognitively able than adults in SNFs or dementia care communities. Those who live or stay in SNFs are usually there for short-term rehabilitation or are almost entirely physically dependent on others for care. Sometimes, in the last stages of dementia, as they become more physically dependent, residents will move from dementia care to an SNF. More often, however, they will live in the dementia care community until death. Before choosing a dementia care community, ask the community's administrator what happens as residents progress in their dementia. Do most residents pass away at the community? Are hospice and palliative care programs allowed to come in and assist in resident care? These important questions will help you learn more about a dementia care community's policies, procedures, and assistance as a loved one is dying.

Depending on their management and location, dementia care communities are often locked, and residents cannot leave the community without assistance. This may seem intimidating at first, but it's for the residents' safety. People with dementia sometimes attempt to "go home" or "go outside" and end up getting lost. Residents are able to go outside the community when a friend, family member, or staff member accompanies them. Some communities also have a center courtyard where residents can come and go as they please.

Continuing-care retirement communities (CCRCs) have multiple levels, such as independent living, assisted living, and skilled nursing. For example, your family member or friend could move from independent living to assisted living and then into a CCRC's dementia care community. One great thing about CCRCs is that your aging parent, partner, or friend is guaranteed a spot in the next level of community care. If you suspect that she will need multiple levels of care, make certain to check whether the communities you visit are CCRCs.

Mary had had dementia for a while, but she had only recently become what is called an "elopement risk." An elopement risk means that a person with dementia is likely to try to leave the community without assistance. Mary also began to withdraw socially in the assisted-living community where she lived. She had trouble making friends as her dementia progressed because none of the other residents at the facility had dementia. Sadly, some of the residents made fun of her because of her trouble speaking and following a conversation. She was distressed and isolated, so her family took her to the dementia care building next door.

Mary improved significantly after moving. She made new friends and began engaging in new pastimes. Suddenly, she was able to participate in activities at her level. She baked cookies, put puzzles together, went out to lunch, and enjoyed singing in groups.

Dementia care communities, like most long-term-care communities, are staffed 24 hours a day, seven days a week. Usually, three shifts of employees and staff members care for residents around the clock. Typically, managerial staff are on-site during normal business hours, so if you have an important question, try to find someone on your family member or friend's management team from 9:00 a.m to 5:00 p.m.

Before choosing a dementia care community, visit the community and learn what services and care it offers. You may want to ask yourself and staff at the community the following questions:

- What are the programs and activities for the residents?
- Does the community host family gatherings or support groups?
- How is the food provided, and can I sample it? Does the community provide snacks between meals?
- What does the community look like? Are there community areas that will provide comfort to your parent, friend, or partner? For example, some communities have a "baby station" with realistic-looking baby dolls, bottles, and baby clothes. Many residents love cuddling and talking to the dolls.
- Are there safe areas where the residents can sit outdoors while remaining within the walls of the community?
- Do the people who work there seem helpful and kind?
- How do the other residents look? Do they look well groomed and healthy? Are any of them close to your friend or family member's level of need? For example, you would not want to move your mother with mild dementia into a community where the other residents are more progressed in dementia and cannot speak or engage with her.

- Will your family member live in a single-occupancy room or a double-occupancy room? If a double, with whom will he share it?
- About how much will it cost per month for your family member's care? Does the community accept Medicaid?
- Are hospice programs allowed to assist with a resident's care? What end-of-life care choices do they offer families?
- What happens if a family runs out of money before their family member passes away? Is financial assistance available, or will the community force the person with dementia to move out?

Make every effort to visit the community twice before making a decision. Try going at different times and on different days, but be aware that residents usually grow more agitated later in the afternoon. Many people with dementia experience *sundowning*, becoming more anxious, fearful, or upset as the day progresses. This topic is covered in more detail in a later chapter.

Talk with residents' family members to get a good feel for the community. Ask others about their experiences and learn what they like and dislike about the community. You can also learn much by watching staff interact with the residents. Do the staff members seem to really know and care about each person? Do they attend to residents quickly and with familiarity? When the staff speak to residents, do they talk at them or with them?

As a caregiver, you may feel anxious about moving your parent, partner, adult child, or friend into a dementia care community. Many family members also feel guilty choosing dementia care because they feel as if someone else is caring for their relative. "I should have taken care of my mom at home," an adult child will say. Many family members are reluctant to leave their parent or partner at a care community, especially for the first time. Choosing the right care community will help ease this guilt.

Your family member or friend with dementia may need a type of care that differs completely from what someone else needs. For some families, in-home care works best, but for others, dementia care communities are better options. As long as you are providing your family member or friend with the best physical and emotional care you can manage, you are doing the right thing. Don't let anyone make you feel as if you have taken the "easy way out" by choosing a dementia care community. You still have to cope with a lot of challenging behaviors, emotions, and concerns when it comes to your family member's care.

2

What Is Dementia?

Dementia describes the loss of cognitive, or thinking or reasoning, function over time. Dementia is an "umbrella" term because it encompasses a large category of diseases. For example, if you find out that a person you know has cancer, you'll probably ask, "What type of cancer?" Cancer includes a large list of potential cancers. Similarly, dementia can result from various diseases. It is not a part of normal aging. Many people know older adults who are "sharp as a tack." Although dementia is a real concern, it is not inevitable.

Many assume the worst when they hear a diagnosis of dementia. Before making any assumptions, however, it is important to know what type of dementia has been diagnosed. Unfortunately, dementia is difficult to fully define. Many with dementia lack an official diagnosis about what has caused the cognitive impairment. Often, someone will say, "My mom has dementia" and leave it at that.

Dementia has more than 70 different causes, and many have important differences in symptoms and in the course of the disease. Some of these causes are reversible (for example, operable brain tumors), so it is imperative that your family member or friend receives a full medical workup. All dementias affect your parent, partner, or friend's ability to function both physically and mentally over time. Someone with dementia could have Alzheimer's disease, frontotemporal lobar dementia, dementia with Lewy bodies, Korsakoff's syndrome (now known as *amnestic syndrome*), Huntington's disease, or another form of cognitive decline, like traumatic brain injury.

You may hear people ask, "What is the difference between Alzheimer's and dementia?" To be clear, Alzheimer's *is* dementia. Alzheimer's disease is the most common form of cognitive decline in older adults, so it gets more attention than other dementias. A person could also have Alzheimer's disease and another type of dementia as well. Although it is confusing, all types of dementia cause cognitive decline and therefore fall under the umbrella term of dementia (see the figure below).

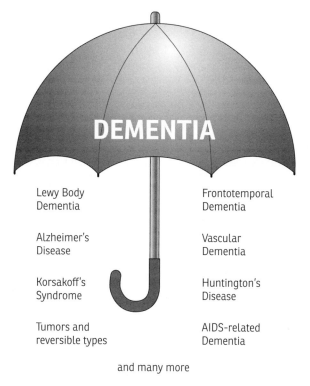

DEMENTIA

Lewy Body
Dementia

Alzheimer's
Disease

Korsakoff's
Syndrome

Tumors and
reversible types

Frontotemporal
Dementia

Vascular
Dementia

Huntington's
Disease

AIDS-related
Dementia

and many more

"Dementia" is an umbrella term for many different diseases that have somewhat different, but related, symptoms.

SYMPTOMS OF DEMENTIA

Cognitive decline encompasses a number of different symptoms. One misconception about dementia is that people who have it always encounter memory-related issues. This isn't always true. The symptoms people have will depend on their type of dementia. Although people with Alzheimer's disease always have memory problems, people with frontotemporal lobar dementia may not have obvious memory deficiencies until much later in the progression of the disease. So a person could have dementia but show no memory challenges at all. People with dementia may have difficulty with the *activities of daily living* (ADLs), such as bathing, dressing, toileting, eating, or walking. They may have trouble with more challenging tasks, such as sending an e-mail or writing a check. These complex tasks are usually referred to as *instrumental activities of daily living*, or IADLs. Sometimes a person with dementia will experience personality changes, sudden mood swings, or even hallucinations. The types of cognitive decline that people with dementia encounter are wide and varied. Unless it is a reversible type, such as from a brain tumor, dementia will eventually lead to death. Although different dementias affect the brain in different ways, all slowly damage the organ until it stops working entirely, and the body shuts down. Often, you'll hear of someone who has dementia dying because of a choking incident or a seemingly unrelated accident like a fall. Although these causes of death are common, dementia probably played a large role in bringing them about. Dementia contributes to death from incidents and accidents, and unless the person passes away from cancer or heart disease, dementia is very often the ultimate cause of death.

What Type of Dementia Is It, and Why Does It Matter?

Many doctors cannot provide a complete diagnosis to their patients with dementia. Because an autopsy is necessary to diagnose a specific type of dementia with 100 percent accuracy, doctors, pathologists, and brain specialists usually offer only a "best guess" as to the cause. "Dementia" is the sole diagnosis for many people moving into a dementia care community. This simply is not enough information for the family or the community. In order to best predict a person's symptoms and care needs, it is important to have a complete and accurate diagnosis.

Although the care and treatment for someone with Alzheimer's disease, for example, may vary little from that for someone with vascular dementia, the symptoms, life span, and causes can differ greatly. Or, someone with frontotemporal lobar dementia may behave in erratic or odd ways. An accurate diagnosis can let you know what to expect. You'll also want to know what type of dementia your parent, partner, or friend has before moving her into a dementia care community. The average care-community resident is in her eighties; female; has Alzheimer's disease; and uses a walker, cane, or wheelchair to get around. If your loved one has frontotemporal lobar dementia, is in her late fifties, and can walk without aid, she may not be a good fit for certain care communities.

ALZHEIMER'S DISEASE

Alzheimer's disease is the most common cause of dementia. People with Alzheimer's disease can live up to 15 or even 20 years after diagnosis but on average live 8 to 11 years. Major symptoms of Alzheimer's disease include forgetfulness, trouble with language, mood changes, issues with visual and depth perception, impaired thinking, and apathy. Like other dementias, as this disease progresses people lose their ability to perform most of the activities of daily living: walking, eating, bathing, and even using the bathroom independently.[1]

Alzheimer's disease doesn't discriminate—it affects people of every background, ethnicity, and sex. However, it *does* disproportionally affect older adults. A person's risk for Alzheimer's increases with age. Alzheimer's is most common in women over the age of 65. Women usually dominate long-term-care communities because women generally live longer than men.[2]

Early-onset Alzheimer's disease is a specific type of dementia that differs from normal Alzheimer's disease. It's a rare but truly heartbreaking disease that affects people younger than age 65. Early-onset Alzheimer's disease is extremely heritable, which means that if one of your parents had it, you are significantly more likely to get it, too. Early-onset Alzheimer's impairs people at a much faster rate than later-onset Alzheimer's.[3] This disease presents a challenge for families looking into dementia care communities because their parent or spouse is usually much younger than the average individual in the community.

Experts have developed a number of tools to help caregivers of people with Alzheimer's or early-onset Alzheimer's (or other types of dementias, for that matter) better understand the disease's stages. Some scales use numbers, while other scales just range from mild to advanced dementia. You may find it challenging to figure out which stage your family member or friend is in, however, because two people with Alzheimer's disease can experience the disease very differently. For example, one 80-year-old woman with Alzheimer's may stay in an advanced stage of dementia for four years. Another woman of the same age may spend five months in a moderate stage before suddenly becoming more advanced in her dementia and passing away. A person with Alzheimer's does not have to cycle through all of the stages before death. She may skip stages or seem to "jump around" from stage to stage.

Vera had Alzheimer's disease. She was in a moderate stage and was incredibly pleasant, funny, and talkative. Despite her cognitive loss, Vera retained much of her positive, happy personality. Every so often, however, she would suddenly become very stubborn and angry. The mood would pass quickly, though, and she would go back to being her joyful self.

Vera didn't realize that her short-term memory was impaired, even though she often asked the same question numerous times within the course of a 10-minute conversation. She was also very physically healthy, other than the Alzheimer's, for a woman of 92.

As we drove down the street in our community van, Vera pointed to a water tower near her old house. "My son climbed that tower when he was a little boy," she said, shaking her head. "I walked outside and saw him halfway up there! I yelled at him, 'You come down this instant!' Oh boy, were his father and I angry at him!" She laughed. Vera's long-term memory was still in very good shape, but she told us this story another five times before we got back to the community.

FRONTOTEMPORAL LOBAR DEMENTIA

What is typically referred to as *frontotemporal lobar dementia* (FTD) or *frontotemporal dementia* is actually a group of diseases. FTD consists of three main types of dementia: behavioral variant FTD (BvFTD), FTD language disorders, and FTD movement disorders. FTD accounts for 10 to 15 percent of all dementias but up to 50 percent of dementias in people under 65 years old. FTD differs from other types of dementia because it affects a younger age group. FTD also presents some significant behavioral, language, and movement challenges that are less prevalent in other dementias.[4]

FTD affects a particular part of the brain: the frontal and temporal lobes. Your *frontal lobe* is the part of your brain that controls decision making and your "filter." This filter is what prevents you from speaking out of turn, making risky choices, or telling your boss what you really think of her.

People with FTD do not experience the memory loss common to Alzheimer's disease—at least not in the beginning of the disease. Typically, family members of a person with FTD will notice their parent, partner, or child acting strangely and take him to see a doctor. The first noticeable changes in a person with FTD are often related to mood, judgment, and impulse control.[5]

Because frontotemporal dementia is a group of diseases, people may experience any of a number of different variations. Budson and Kowall, in their 2014 book *The Handbook of Alzheimer's Disease and Other Dementias*, suggest that people with BvFTD experience an odd set of behavioral changes that can make long-term dementia caregiving uniquely challenging.[6] Because it affects people who are in their forties or fifties, others often fail to realize that their parent, partner, child, or friend is experiencing dementia-related symptoms. Sometimes, odd behaviors may even get written off as a "midlife crisis" because they are so out of character for the individual with FTD. Difficulties making plans, an inability to control impulses, a loss of inhibition, social awkwardness, passivity, inappropriate sexual comments or actions, and cravings for sweets are all common among people with BvFTD. A good example of this disorder is the man who had a great relationship with his wife until his late forties. Suddenly, he began cheating on her—and told everyone about it. Not only was it out of character for him, it was an alarming change from his past behavior. The man was unaware of his sudden personality change, but his wife was acutely aware of it and took him to a neurologist, who diagnosed him with FTD.

FTD language disorders affect a person's ability to speak normally. Even the most eloquent of speakers, if afflicted with FTD, can lose his ability to make sense when speaking—or even lose the ability to speak entirely. Words become jumbled, terms become broad (saying "the thing" or "it" instead of clarifying), and even the ability to understand language declines.

In FTD movement disorders, automatic muscle functions become impaired. People with FTD may experience tremors and spasms or even difficulty walking and balancing.[7]

People with FTD can find dementia care communities difficult environments to live in. Most residents are at least a decade older than a person with FTD. When these older residents listen to music, watch movies, or talk about the past, they are not referring to the recent past that someone with FTD may relate to. A person with FTD may not fare well in a dementia care community until he is much more progressed in the disease.

Nicholas was excited that he and his wife, Janice, were getting a new floor in their kitchen. They had just begun talking about the process and needed to save up some money before hiring a contractor. Janice told Nicholas that it would probably be another six months before they would be able to start getting a new floor.

One day Janice came home to find that Nick had ripped up the entire kitchen floor—without any warning. He had come home from work, decided it was time, and begun taking apart the floorboards. The couple had to live with this change for months before they could afford to hire someone to fix it.

Nicholas was eventually diagnosed with BvFTD. His inability to make decisions, process information, and self-monitor had caused him to rip the floor up long before the couple was able to pay for it. He had no sense of why this behavior was bizarre or alarming because the filter part of his brain was not working properly.

VASCULAR DEMENTIA

Strokes or other blood vessel damage in the brain can lead to various types of vascular dementia (VaD). VaD is sometimes known as *vascular cognitive impairment*, or VCI, to show that it is actually a group of dementias related to cerebrovascular damage. Someone with VaD will usually have trouble with shape discrimination, object perception, and spatial awareness. He will also tend to have difficulties with motor coordination and reflex speed. Vascular dementia affects the way a person walks, sometimes described as a *gait disturbance*. Although these symptoms can seem almost normal after a person suffers a stroke, they could be signs of VaD. Of course, like most dementias, a person with VaD typically will also have trouble with memory, especially later in the disease.

VaD is often called "the preventable dementia" because people who stay relatively healthy and avoid arteriosclerosis, hypertension, diabetes, smoking, and obesity are unlikely to get it. That being said, it is still one of the most common forms of dementia worldwide, second only to Alzheimer's disease.[8]

Karen could still play the piano, but she played it entirely from memory—not from the book sitting on the piano stand. Karen flipped the book's pages as if she were reading the music, but the pages never matched the song she actually played. In fact, she only had about five songs that she would play over and over again.

Her memory, especially early in VaD, was not that poor. She could remember people she had just met, play those piano songs from memory, and keep track of time during the day. Karen's recall and processing declined over time, but her walk and spatial awareness grew worse than her memory. She had difficulty discriminating between open and closed doors. She also had issues opening closed doors. Patterns on the carpet confused her. If a carpet had a line on it, Karen would step over the line. She also seemed to have trouble walking, although she did not use a cane or walker. Her arms stayed locked at her sides as she shuffled down the hallways. It almost seemed as though her knees refused to bend. Still, Karen took no notice of this problem.

DEMENTIA WITH LEWY BODIES

Lewy body–related diseases account for 10 percent to 25 percent of all dementias. Three different diseases comprise this group: dementia with Lewy bodies (DLB), Parkinson's disease dementia, and Parkinson's disease. Parkinson's disease is a type of Lewy body disease, but you can have it without having dementia. You can, however, have Parkinson's disease dementia, in which dementia symptoms manifest shortly after a Parkinson's diagnosis. People who have DLB may have some Parkinsonian symptoms, but they don't have full-blown Parkinson's.[9]

A few symptoms set DLB apart from Alzheimer's disease and other dementias. For one, people with DLB tend to hallucinate. Strange, complex paranoias can accompany these vivid visual hallucinations. Although people with other dementias can hallucinate, it's very rare. If you notice that your family member or friend is hallucinating and she hasn't experienced it before, immediately take her to a doctor. If it's a common occurrence, however, do not make the experience of hallucinating even scarier for her: make sure to agree with what she is seeing.[10]

Other symptoms that set these dementias apart from others include sleep-related disorders; Parkinson's symptoms such as tremors or slow, rigid movements; and *fluctuating impairment*. People with fluctuating impairment may seem very different from one day to the next. Their attention and alertness may vary.

OTHER DEMENTIAS

More than 70 different conditions cause dementia. While Alzheimer's disease, VaD, DLB, and FTD are the most common, a person with dementia could have one or even several different diagnoses. It's incredibly important that your family member or friend receives a full medical workup when diagnosing dementia. A brain tumor, for example, can cause a potentially reversible type of dementia. Without a full checkup, doctors could easily mistake it for Alzheimer's disease, which has a different course of treatment.[11]

One type of dementia that receives little attention happens as a result of a traumatic brain injury (TBI). TBI is very serious and often occurs after a major accident or even a significant number of concussions.

William was not the normal dementia patient. At only 65 years old, William had already experienced significant cognitive decline. In his senior year of high school, he received a full football scholarship to college. William played well his first few years in college, but he received many concussions. The coaches benched William, telling him it was too dangerous for him to continue playing the game he loved. William transferred to a smaller school and left his scholarship behind. He continued to play football and suffered more and more concussions. William then graduated and worked for many years. Eventually, however, the past caught up with him.

Now, he sat in our lobby waiting for a nurse to see him. "I don't belong in here," he argued. "Why are all these old people in this place!" It was sad, but William was right—he was not like everyone else. Because he had decided to continue playing football, William actually gave himself dementia early in life. In fact, William's own father—a man of 92 years old—was William's main caregiver.

DELIRIUM

Delirium causes a rapid and sudden onset of confusion and change in alertness. Delirium is *not* dementia, which is marked by a slow and progressive decline. If your family member or friend acted normal 10 minutes earlier and then suddenly seems to be in a "fog" or acts very confused or aggressive, you'll want to get her evaluated for the cause. Many people with dementia get delirium after surgery, new medicine, or urinary tract infections (UTIs), so it is important to check with a doctor when noticeable changes occur.[12]

Brian was admitted to the hospital for emergency retina surgery. At 56, he'd had a few eye surgeries but never any other real medical problems. He was generally healthy, active, and intelligent. The surgeons anesthetized him for the procedure so that he would not be awake during surgery.

After the procedure, which went well, Brian woke up sick and exhausted. His stomach hurt, he had a headache, and of course, his eye felt beaten and bruised. He returned home to rest and recover.

For about two weeks after the surgery, Brian felt odd. He was confused, disorganized, and easily distracted. His wife had trouble holding a conversation with him. Brian also found that he would leave a room, head to another, and have no idea why he had gone to the new space. The anesthesia and bodily stress from the surgery had caused Brian's delirium. Because it was reversible, after some time the confusion began to fade.

Aware of the challenges he was experiencing, Brian probably should have seen a physician. Although his delirium resolved, other, potentially more dangerous conditions could have caused his confusion.

No matter what type of dementia your parent, partner, child, or friend has, you will undoubtedly encounter many of the physical and psychological changes listed in this chapter. It is imperative to make sure that he sees a physician on a regular basis. It is also important to keep track of changes over time. You know this person better than anyone, so don't be afraid to seek a second, or even a third, opinion from doctors when it comes to his care.

4

When It's Time for a Dementia Care Community— and When It's Not

Moving your parent, partner, or adult child into a dementia care community will be a big change for you and your family, so make sure you are doing it for the right reasons—and at the right time. Perhaps you are struggling with your family member's 24-hour needs. The physical and emotional demands of caregiving are weighing on you and your own independence. You may discover that a care community is the right choice.

PHYSICAL NEEDS

As a person's dementia progresses, her family may become unable to care for her physically. This is one of the most common reasons for placing a loved one in a dementia care community. When your parent, partner, child, or friend with dementia requires assistance to walk, eat, and bathe, her needs can become overwhelming. You should not strain your body attempting to move or transfer her. In a dementia care community the staff can work together—and often do—to assist residents.

Incontinence is also an issue for individuals with moderate to advanced dementia. Urinary or bowel incontinence means that a person loses control over her bladder and bowel functions. People with dementia will eventually require disposable adult briefs made for incontinence and need frequent changing. Incontinence can be incredibly challenging—and potentially embarrassing—for family caregivers to handle. Trained, experienced staff members at dementia care communities are comfortable coping with incontinence in their residents.

EMOTIONAL NEEDS

Families may consider dementia care communities when they feel emotionally unable to continue caring for a parent, partner, or child with dementia. Caring for another person is incredibly challenging and stressful. Caregivers have lives to live, too, and a number of other responsibilities. Caring for a loved one with dementia is a full-time, unpaid job—and many caregivers *already* have a full-time day job.

Recognize that taking your family member or friend to a care community is not neglecting him; in fact, it will probably improve your relationship with him. Consider this: When you're constantly caring for your father, you get caught up in the stressful, day-to-day tasks and physical needs that he requires. It's not uncommon for family caregivers to lament about how physically exhausting the hands-on care can become. When you visit your father in a dementia care community, the 24-hour staff have already met his physical needs. You are able to provide emotional support for your father without worrying about the hands-on care.

Perhaps you are trying an in-home-care agency, but the help it has provided you in caring for your father 24 hours a day has been inadequate. It's been difficult to schedule caregivers, and when they do get scheduled, they cancel or quit at the last minute. At a dementia care community, your father will receive daily care regardless of what staff members call in sick or quit. You'll no longer have to worry about the schedules of home-care agency workers.

SAFETY CONCERNS

One of the biggest reasons for placing a family member or friend in a dementia care community is because that person is "wandering."

Families often have trouble keeping someone with dementia safe, especially when that person lives at home. Even in the early stages of dementia, people will get lost in familiar places. Some people in the later stages of dementia will walk constantly, often picking up objects on the way that seem interesting to them. People in these stages are particularly concerning because many cannot verbalize who they are or where they live. If they get lost outside, they may not be able to ask for help. If a person with dementia lives at home, it is imperative to lock the doors so he cannot exit without the aid of a caregiver. Some companies sell door locks made specifically for this situation.

Even with an in-home-care agency, your house may not be the best place for your parent, partner, child, or friend with dementia. Floor mats or rugs can be slip hazards, stairs can cause dangerous falls, and even appliances such as the stove or toaster oven can be hazardous. Although your family member or friend may feel as though she can do everything she always did, you know this isn't the case. Your mother once enjoyed baking cookies by herself, but she may now forget she left the oven on. As dementia-proof as you make your house, it will never be as safe as a community designed for people with cognitive loss.

ASSISTED LIVING

Maybe your family member or friend is living in an independent- or assisted-living community. Recall that these communities typically don't keep the doors locked 24 hours a day. Residents with dementia may not only be unsafe in one of these communities, but they may also withdraw socially. Whether your parent, partner, child, or friend lives at home alone or in a community surrounded by people, it is possible that she will lose the capacity to engage with others who are not on her cognitive level. Some people with dementia start withdrawing socially because they become aware of their limitations and feel embarrassed. Others withdraw out of necessity: perhaps the types of activities and programs available make no sense to them.

Unfortunately, some people in assisted living, whether out of fear or cruelty, may actually tease or socially isolate people with dementia. In cases like these, it may be best to consider a dementia care community. The residents in many dementia care communities enjoy each other's company. They also enjoy the ability to engage in activities designed specifically for their needs. Many dementia-specific communities offer easy-to-complete activities for their residents. For example, while one resident works on a puzzle, another may sort and fold socks, while still another could arrange flowers or type on a community computer. It is uncommon to find that kind of hands-on, strategic programming in most assisted-living communities because the residents simply don't need it.

For a number of reasons, you may want to try a dementia care community for your family member's care. Be it out of physical or emotional necessity, safety, or social requirements, your parent, partner, child, sibling, or friend could benefit from 24-hour dementia care within a community.

"Mom wants to live at home where she has always lived," Sally said. "She loves it here; it just wouldn't be fair to relocate her." Sally spent a lot of time searching the Internet for potential caregivers. In fact, she hired three shifts of caregivers—every day.

I spent two nights each week looking after Sally's 90-year-old mother, Margaret. Margaret, in a moderate stage of Alzheimer's disease, would wake up frequently throughout the night to use the bathroom. I slept in Margaret's quiet old house and woke up regularly to the sound of a motion alarm, signaling that she had gotten out of bed. I would help Margaret walk to the bathroom and use the toilet and then get her back to bed.

The more time I spent with Margaret, the more I realized that Sally was incorrect about her mother's feelings toward the house: In truth, Margaret had no idea that she still lived at home. "I had better call my husband," she would tell me. "I need to let him know that I'm staying at this hotel tonight."

Margaret didn't realize that it was her house because the people she loved no longer lived there. A house is not a home unless it contains things that connect a person to it emotionally, and for Margaret, those things were not there. Margaret's husband had passed away, and her children were adults. Still, Margaret's family remained convinced that it would be cruel to move her into a dementia care community, even as they struggled to find caregivers to look after her around the clock. She often asked to "go home" even though she had lived in the house for more than 50 years. In truth, Margaret was a perfect candidate for a dementia care community and would never have even realized that she was living in one.

WHEN IT'S *NOT* TIME FOR A DEMENTIA CARE COMMUNITY

The decision to take your parent, partner, child, or sibling to a dementia care community is personal. With that said, in some instances your family member with dementia will not be a good fit for a dementia care community.

Should My Loved One Be in an Assisted-Living Community?

Sometimes, an assisted-living community is better for a person with mild dementia. Although most residents in assisted-living communities do not have dementia, some residents do have mild cognitive impairment or mild dementia.

Charlie was moved into a dementia care community well before he was ready for the level of care it provided. His dementia symptoms were mild, and he was not ready to live in a community locked 24 hours a day. Charlie stayed in his room constantly. He refused to engage in any programs because he was afraid of the other residents.

"I'm sorry," he said. "I'm just afraid to talk to anyone here. Sometimes a woman walks in my room and just starts going on and on about things I don't understand. Why is she acting like that?" Although he wanted to make new friends, he was unable to find anyone at his cognitive level. While other residents happily engaged with one another, Charlie was an outcast. Eventually, Charlie moved into a nearby assisted-living community.

Most residents living in dementia care communities do very well and benefit from positively interacting with others. And, for the most part, even the higher-functioning residents do not realize that there is anything abnormal about others who live in the community. But when a resident is frightened of other people in the community or believes they are "crazy," he is *not* a good fit for a dementia-specific unit.

A doctor may occasionally suggest dementia community placement for a person who isn't yet ready for it. Overall, you need to know your family member's level of dementia to decide when a dementia care community is appropriate. Recognize that some communities will have higher-functioning residents than others and may offer different levels of activities. Visit your local dementia-specific communities to decide what is best for your parent, partner, child, or sibling. You'll know almost immediately if there are residents at each one with whom he will be able to interact.

Should My Loved One Be in a Skilled-Nursing Facility?

Your family member may need more care than a dementia care community typically provides. Skilled-nursing facilities, or SNFs, are typically for residents who require complete, or nearly complete, physical assistance. For example, if your mother uses a wheelchair, needs to be fed, cannot be transferred to a bed or a toilet without at least two people's assistance, and is completely incontinent, she may be a good fit for an SNF. Sadly, some family members wait too long to choose a dementia care community. By the time they decide on one, the person with dementia is a better candidate for an SNF. People with very advanced dementia don't typically benefit from the activities and resident interaction that occur in dementia care communities. When deciding if a dementia care community is right for your mother, for example, ask yourself some important questions:

- Is your mother able to interact with others? Will she be able to make friends at a dementia care community? If she has trouble communicating or understanding people, she may fare better at an SNF.
- Have you talked to the nurse or director at your local dementia-specific community? He or she may be able to tell you if the community has other residents with the same physical needs as your mother.
- Will your mother enjoy performers and group activities? If so, she should be in a dementia care community.
- What are the costs associated with each community? Is a dementia care community more expensive? Will your mother get enough positive interaction from an SNF? Although cost is important, it's also necessary to weigh the benefits your mother will get from living in a more connected community.

If your mother would have a better life at a dementia-specific community, you should choose that as her new home. Visit a few communities in order to get a feel for the environment they provide. Above all, trust your gut feeling.

Wherever you choose to move your parent, partner, child, or sibling, don't get discouraged if she doesn't immediately "fit in." Even though she may ask to go home or complain about other residents, give her time to get used to the community. It is important for family members to recognize that many residents take a week or two to fully adjust to a new environment.

5

Caring for People Is an Imperfect Science

Staff at long-term care communities do their best to do the right thing by their residents. Still, try as they might, some things just don't go as planned. Falls, accidents, scheduling conflicts with staff members, and even power outages all occur. There are missed snack times, lost shoes, entertainers that cancel, and confusing care plans. Any good care community will do its best to work with you when you or your family have a complaint or question. Some days, though, nothing goes right.

My phone began ringing at about 10:00 a.m., and it did not stop until about 5:00 p.m. I wasn't even at work that day, for I had taken a paid time-off day for a small family vacation. That did not stop the calls, texts, and e-mails. I was immediately emotionally engaged in the whole situation. Everything that could have gone wrong over the weekend seemed to have gone wrong. Some staff called in sick, a couple of residents died, a computer system crashed, and one family became very angry.

"My mom's shoes are missing," Tonya yelled at me over the phone. "Why does this keep happening? You tell me that a resident takes them, but that is ridiculous! Can't you pay more attention to these residents?"

I tried to calm Tonya down and explain that this was just a misunderstanding—and that I could really do nothing from my car.

I don't write that story to ask you to feel sorry for my situation or even to think twice before calling a manager at your family member or friend's community for help. I simply want to illustrate that although we try our best, things do go wrong. Caring for people is an imperfect science. Looking after older adults with dementia is even more imperfect. The people employed in long-term-care communities work very hard. They are generally not paid nearly as well as they should be. Still, everyone gives their all to care for older adults who need assistance. Sometimes, a simple "thank you" goes a long way when talking to the hands-on caregivers at a care community.

The residents of care communities have varying needs, backgrounds, and care plans. Although any good care community will do its best to take the weight off you and your family, sometimes it will fail to meet your expectations. Like any business, many pieces go into making a care community run effectively. Everyone has a boss—even the leader at your family member or friend's care community. And occasionally, these business-like power dynamics make dementia care communities even more confusing.

THE EXECUTIVE DIRECTOR

The executive director is the person who runs your parent, partner, child, or friend's community on a day-to-day basis. Some communities also have an associate or assistant executive director who serves as the executive director's right hand. It is imperative that you meet—and like—the director at your family member's community. This person usually has a lot of say about the way the community is run, and he or she can really change the work ethic and vibe around the facility. Typically, however, this person and his or her staff answer to a regional team, or a few regional members, who do not normally work at the facility. The regional team probably oversees the community from a larger perspective. The bigger the senior living company is, the more regional people will work there. This team manages everything from finances to big-picture nursing care. When it comes to big decisions, such as whether to accept a challenging resident into the community, regional teams are very influential.

OTHER POSITIONS

Each community will have similar positions, but their names for those positions may differ. Most places will have one or more nurses (depending on the size of the community), an activity director, a dietary director or lead chef, a few maintenance workers, housekeepers, a business office manager, one or two marketing directors, and potentially a few other management positions. All of these positions work both independently and as a team to make sure the community runs as well as it can. For a business that runs 24 hours a day, seven days a week, communication between families and management becomes very important. The best way to communicate with a community's management team is to find one or two managers who can assist you directly. For example, if your family member or friend is on a specific floor, look for the nurse or manager of that floor. Find that person's phone number and e-mail address so that you can speak to her directly.

STAFFING ISSUES

Most dementia-specific communities will have at least three shifts of workers throughout the day. Although necessary, this brings its own issues. Inevitably, communication errors and missed messages will happen regarding resident care. Because so many employees work in any given long-term-care community, a message has multiple chances to get lost. For example, a family member may ask a manager to ensure that third-shift workers clean his mother's room. Perhaps that manager didn't stay late enough and forgot to write a note to third shift, or perhaps a staff member called in sick, and the staff on third shift did not get the memo. Suddenly, the room does not get cleaned, despite everyone's best intentions. A mixed or missed message is probably one of the biggest causes of confusion or mistakes in long-term care.

Long-term-care communities are notorious for high staff-turnover rates. The hands-on caregivers, in particular, are typically underpaid. They quit often and are replaced very quickly. Even at the managerial level, it seems as though people get traded between companies frequently. Even the best communities gain and lose staff members quickly, so training and rehiring are always going on. This, in and of itself, causes some confusion throughout any care community.

THE BENEFITS

Despite the things that can go wrong during your family member or friend's stay at a care community, the benefits of choosing long-term care often far outweigh the negatives. You, as a caregiver, will be free of the weight of having to provide for your parent, partner, adult child, or friend 24 hours a day. You know that, no matter what, he is receiving care. He is with people who are at the same cognitive level and have similar needs. He has the ability to make friends and eat well-balanced meals every day. Caring for people is an imperfect science, and things won't always go as planned. Despite this, a care community can provide a wonderful opportunity for your family member or friend to thrive.

PART II

COMMUNICATING WITH SOMEONE WHO HAS DEMENTIA

6

Embrace Their Reality:
When Loved Ones Are Confused

When caring for someone with dementia, you'll quickly come to learn that his reality is not the same as yours. This person may tell you many things that are not true, even things that are completely impossible. This is because dementia often robs the person of his ability to recall information the same way he used to. When someone with dementia hears new information, it doesn't stay in his memory. What does remain is old information, including things he heard, learned, or experienced decades earlier. Sometimes, when you hear something confusing from a person with dementia, it's because he is mixing up the past, present, and future—the ability to understand time is no longer flawless. Rather than resisting the person's reality, embrace that reality, and you'll likely find that your acceptance of his changed perceptions will make all the difference in your relationship.

"Embracing someone's reality" may sometimes make you feel as if you're lying. From a young age, parents teach their children that lying is wrong. Incorrect statements should be corrected, and untruths should not be said. Why, then, do I advise going along with a story from someone who has dementia when the story does not make sense or appears untruthful? This example illustrates how embracing someone's reality can lead to a better outcome for the person with dementia and those around him:

I once overheard a nurse arguing with a man who had dementia. He was irate and banging on the door to another resident's room. "That's my wife!" he yelled. "My wife is in there, and you better let me in to see her!"

"That is not your wife," the nurse said. "You cannot come in here while we are getting her changed." The more she told him this, the more frustrated and angry he became.

"That is my wife. That's my wife. Let me in there! You think I don't know what my wife looks like?" he shouted, slamming his walker into the door. This resident wasn't his wife, but telling him so wasn't helping the situation.

I walked up and laid my hand on his shoulder. "Hey, let's wait out here for her. She'll be ready soon," I assured him. He calmed down immediately and sat with me. I looked to the nurse and suggested she avoid arguing with him. She became defensive and said she did not want to lie to him.

This is a typical response. Caregivers want to do the "right" thing, especially if caring for a parent or spouse. Many caregivers ask me: Is "lying" really the best option? They have spent their whole lives being truthful with their loved ones, so why should they stop now?

REDIRECTION AND DISTRACTION

Several techniques are useful when interacting with a person who has dementia. One is *redirection*, which redirects your family member to a safer, more acceptable activity. For example, if your father tries to shave with a straight razor, provide an electric razor instead. It is safer and easier for him to manage. You can also redirect by changing the conversation to a more positive topic. If a man with dementia wants to go visit his mother, for example, you could ask him what he loves most about her and therefore avoid distressing him.

Another option, *distraction*, involves completely changing the action or activity. For example, if your father is crying because he cannot find his parents, ask him to help you prepare dinner. This gives him something enjoyable to do, and he will likely forget his worry. Does the following scenario sound familiar?

Your 85-year-old mother is looking at the clock. "When are we going to Mom's house?" she asks, although her mother has been deceased for years.

You could react to this in several ways. Sadly, many caregivers take the wrong approach: "Mom, you are 85. Grandma has been dead for 20 years," you might explain, annoyed that she is so confused. But although you may believe this little reminder will be helpful, the information devastates your mother. "When did she die?" she asks, tears in her eyes. Fifteen minutes later, she has forgotten that you've told her this, but she is still upset and agitated and does not know why.

A potentially better solution could be to redirect the conversation. "I'm not sure," you could say in answer to her initial question. "What were you thinking of doing at Mom's house?" Maybe you could remind her of Grandma's cooking and how delicious her sweet potatoes always tasted. She may happily talk about this, and suddenly your negative conversation turns positive.

If that does not work, try distracting her with something else. Although the term "distraction" doesn't sound very dignified, this technique can improve your relationship with a family member or friend who has dementia. "I'm not sure, Mom," you say. "But I really need some help finishing up these dishes. Could you clean off these plates for me?" Now, you have just successfully used two positive strategies for embracing your mother's reality.

WHEN REDIRECTION AND DISTRACTION DON'T WORK

Redirection and distraction are not always effective. For some with dementia, more *embracing* goes a long way. At this point, dementia care can become difficult for some caregivers because this technique can feel like lying. But think about embracing someone's reality as accepting the world in which she lives instead of the world in which you live. Trying to drag someone with dementia back into our world is unfair.

One woman I looked after had to take multiple medications. Each day when I went to check on her, she was convinced that she had already taken her heart medication. "I already took that today," she argued on one such morning. "I took it at 6:00 a.m., and no one was here to see me take it. But I remember taking it, and I am not taking another one."

The pills were still in her pillbox, so she had clearly not taken anything. But she truly believed she had already taken the pills and refused to take them "again," which made sense in her reality.

"Oh, I just called your doctor, and he said you have to take a second dose," I explained, thinking quickly.

"Oh, okay, thank you for calling him!" She smiled, holding out her hand for the pills. This made sense in her reality, and she accepted the first of her medications for the day.

It's important to keep in mind that the reality of a person with dementia is not the same as yours. Such statements aren't lies when someone is so deep in dementia that she cannot comprehend the real truth. Once caregivers understand this, life can be less complicated and hurtful for all involved.

Bella did not want to get off the bus. She had finished her doctor's appointment and had arrived back at our dementia care community, but she didn't understand where she was. "This isn't my house," she said, her voice rising. "I want this bus to take me to my house, where it picked me up!" No matter what I said, Bella remained determined to sit on this bus forever.

"I am not getting off this bus," she argued. "You are trying to trick me. This is not my house, and I want this bus to take me to my house right this instant." Of course, she had not lived alone for years, and we needed to get her off the vehicle. She was far enough into dementia that she was confused about her location but aware enough to argue vehemently that she did not wish to get off the bus.

I had to embrace her reality and understand her situation. I explained that we would need to get on another bus because this bus only took a certain route. She insisted that we move to the next stop. I convinced the bus driver to drive us around for 10 minutes and then park behind the building.

"Okay, we're here!" I said with some enthusiasm when we arrived back at the community. She was not pleased, but I promised that we would only be staying at this "hotel" for a short time. Finally, I was able to coax her off the bus.

I tried multiple tactics to get Bella to follow me off that bus. Eventually, one (or perhaps a combination of techniques) worked. Dementia care has a lot to do with patience but also a lot to do with creativity. Step into your loved one's shoes. Remember that her reality is not the same as your reality anymore. Here are a few steps that can be taken if a person with dementia needs calming or requires help:

1. First, ask him questions and engage him. When someone is crying and looking for his parents, say, "Wow, it sounds like you really miss your parents. Can you tell me more about them?" This uses positive, verbal redirection.
2. If this does not work, try to redirect the person's attention: "Instead of leaving right now to go look for them, could we wait a little while? Come sit with me over here."
3. Try to distract the person. "Dad, I need your help shucking this corn for dinner."
4. If questions, redirection, and distraction don't work, go a little further. Find out where your friend or family member thinks his parents are, and then go from there. If he says, "They always work during the day," you could say, "I think your mom and dad are at work right now. It's not time for them to get off of work yet, but I'm sure they'll come home as soon as they are finished."

Embracing your loved one's reality will make your relationship with him more positive. When visiting a family member in a dementia care community, your time is even more precious than when you were caring for him at home, so it is imperative to keep the interaction as pleasant as possible.

7

Why It Doesn't Work to Reorient People Who Have Dementia

People with dementia do not always live in the same world that we do. Although they may be physically present, their minds are elsewhere. Many older adults with dementia find the past, present, and future very confusing. It's not uncommon for them to believe that their past is their present because their "timeline" is no longer working. For example, your mother may think she is 20 years old and has just entered college. In her mind her grandchildren are her classmates, and she has yet to meet her husband. You find yourself playing along, and that is exactly what you should do. You hesitate, however, because you feel the urge to "tell her the truth" and bring her back to your world. Sometimes, it's difficult to embrace her reality and agree with everything she says, particularly when it makes tasks like taking her to a doctor's appointment very challenging. "But I don't need to go see a doctor," she says. "We have one right here on campus!" Although you want to tell her the truth, recall that it is your job, as her caregiver, to embrace her reality.

In dementia care, there are a few caregiving techniques to always avoid. The terms *orienting* or *reorienting* describe a process in which a caregiver brings the person with dementia back to reality. This is the opposite of embracing someone's reality and has no place in positive dementia care. Statements like "Your parents have been dead for years" or "Your children are adults now" are examples of reorientation. Both of these statements are meant to "correct" a person with dementia, and that tactic is not appropriate. Although it's imperative that we know how to embrace someone's reality, it's also important to know what happens when we do the opposite.

It can be very tempting to "remind" a person with dementia of the truth. Often, families believe this will help the person recall the truth, but this is not always the case. Even if he does remember, the information can confuse or upset him. For example, reminding your father with dementia that his parents are dead, that he lives in a facility, or that it is no longer the decade that he thinks it is can be very cruel. Your dad may seem to recall this information after you have provided it, but he'll be upset that he forgot it in the first place. And after a little while, the facts will leave his mind again. You succeeded in reminding him of the truth, but his foul mood stuck around much longer than the information did. It is a lose-lose situation: neither you nor your dad has gained anything in this exchange.

Consider, also, that a person with dementia often does not realize that the truth contains facts at all. For example, your mother may not recall that she attended her sister's funeral six years earlier. When she asks where her sister is, it is important that you don't bombard her with the truth. By letting her know that her sister is deceased, you are introducing new information into the conversation. In her current reality, your mother is unaware that her sister is deceased, and you just told her, seemingly for the first time. She will no doubt be upset, agitated, and confused. "What else don't I know about?" she may ask herself—and you. When we remind people with dementia of facts they do not remember, we remind them that they have dementia. We remind them that something is wrong with the way they think and feel.

We may also believe that a person with dementia will not remember what we tell him. This can make it tempting to reorient him for a moment. It is important to remember that although a person with dementia may not remember what he has heard, he can still remain confused and upset long after the conversation ends. Emotion has an incredibly strong influence on memory. A painful memory has the ability to stick around much longer than a pleasant one. It is a much simpler—and often happier—approach to just live in that person's reality.

Often, the person with dementia lives in a much happier reality than ours. Recall that in his world, certain things are true: perhaps his parents are alive, or maybe he has a job interview to attend. Reorienting a person with dementia can be a heartbreaking experience for both parties. It is not only improper care—it's also cruel.

Eva sat in the front room of the community, staring hard out the door. It was still early in the morning, so I was surprised to see her there. Although Eva often sat near the door waiting to "go home," she usually did not feel anxious about it until later in the day. As I walked in the door, I approached her chair. "Hey, Eva," I said. "What are you doing here?"

"I just found out that my parents died," Eva explained slowly, tears in her eyes. "One of the girls here just came up and told me that. She said they've been dead for a long time. I cannot believe I missed the funeral. I never got to say goodbye to them." She was heartbroken.

I felt sad for Eva and angry, too. I wasn't sure who had told her this "truth" in an attempt to reorient her. I couldn't say much to help Eva at this point, but I offered my hand. "I don't know why anyone would say that," I said. "But I am so sorry to hear about it. I understand their funeral is tomorrow, so don't worry—you didn't miss it." This was the reassurance that Eva needed.

I was eventually able to calm Eva down and get her to follow me to an activity. She began to enjoy herself and was able to put the anxiety behind her.

Had I handled that situation differently, such as agreeing that Eva's parents had been dead for years, chaos would probably have ensued. Not only had she just learned that her parents were dead, she'd heard that they had actually been gone for years. She probably wondered what she had been doing that whole time and why she had not had the chance to say goodbye. By embracing her reality, I was able to give her closure in her parents' death. Suggesting that they had died years before did not provide closure at all: in fact, it just brought pain.

Embracing a person's reality without reorienting her is key to positive dementia care. Relationships with our loved ones with dementia flourish when we accept that they live in a different world than we do.

The best way to succeed with these methods is to make them fun: What reality does your sister with dementia live in today? Is she 20 years old and still in college? Is she planning a surprise birthday party for your father? If you can find the reality and play along, life with your family member or friend will not only be easier, it will also be more fulfilling. Dementia is a challenging and often upsetting group of diseases. It is easier said than done, but finding the beauty and whimsical parts in your parent, partner, child, sibling, or friend's cognitive loss will keep your relationship from falling on hard times.

8

Why Quizzing Isn't Effective

It is a challenge, at times, to find things to talk about with people who have dementia. We all ask our friends questions such as "What have you been doing today?" or "Where did you go to dinner last night?" Carrying on this type of conversation is often very difficult, however, for people with dementia. Although they can usually talk about their childhood with ease, recalling short-term details and information is nearly impossible. This is why *quizzing*, or asking numerous questions, is a bad way to communicate with a person who has dementia.

Eleanor's grandchildren, now adults in their twenties and thirties, were excited to see their grandmother. They did not, however, know how to navigate Eleanor's Alzheimer's disease. Every time they visited her, they quizzed her about what she had done that day, what she had eaten, and who she had talked to. They were not trying to be unkind—they just weren't sure what to talk to their grandmother about.

"Hi!" one of the young women greeted Eleanor. "Do you remember who I am?"

Eleanor paused, smiling anxiously. "Well, of course! You're . . . you are . . . um . . ." She stumbled over her words, trying to search her brain for the right information.

"I'm Suzanne, your granddaughter!" the woman said, smiling and attempting to be helpful.

"Of course! Yes, Suzanne, I'm sorry. I'm just having such a busy day. You know how those things are," Eleanor offered, trying to understand why she was struggling to recall her own granddaughter's name and face.

It is not uncommon to see family and friends of residents with dementia use questioning and quizzing as a form of conversation. Although finding things to talk about with a person who has dementia isn't easy, quizzing is never the right approach. It is also tempting for family members to test their loved one's memory when they visit. Quizzing will not help a person remember information nor will it prepare her for questions in the future. When someone has dementia, she does not have complete control over her brain's functions. It is unfair to ask her to recall facts, events, or people when she simply lacks the ability to do so.

WHEN VISITING

If you have a family member or friend with dementia, particularly if that person lives in a dementia care community, you may find it tempting to ask her about what she did that day before you arrived. Outside of dementia care, this is normal practice. In dementia care, however, it's not wise to quiz a person about her day. You may receive incorrect information or maybe no information at all.

For example, asking your mother if she went out for ice cream with the rest of the residents, when you know that she did, is a poor choice. You already know the answer, and asking if she remembers puts her in a compromising position. She may not recall going on an outing, even if it ended only an hour ago. She may also become upset or frustrated if she felt as though she missed out. Along the same lines, asking your mother if she had lunch is also not wise—especially if you already know the answer. Many people with dementia do not recall short-term memories, particularly those not attached to emotion. Even if she had fun on the ice cream outing or enjoyed a nice lunch, she may have difficulty figuring out when events happened, especially if they are recurring, like eating lunch. Your mother could be thinking of yesterday's lunch, or even last week's lunch. "No, I didn't eat at all today," she may respond.

As always, it is imperative that you embrace your family member or friend's reality, whatever that reality is. It is okay to ask about her day, but do not expect a perfect answer. Going along with the story will make the experience positive for everyone.

"What have you been up to today?" Hilda's guests asked her.

"Oh, boy, we went for a lovely bike ride through the countryside!" Hilda exclaimed. "It was so beautiful. We all had such a lovely time."

Hilda's guests were clearly puzzled, but they went along with her story. "Oh . . . wow, that sounds . . . that sounds fun," one offered, clearly confused.

Although Hilda had gone on no such bike ride, she believed that she had. In her world, what she had done that morning was completely different than what she had actually been doing. Although her story was not true, it was interesting and fun for her. And, it is important to note, Hilda wasn't lying. Because of her dementia, Hilda's brain had created a fake story that made sense to her. She truly believed she had gone on a bike ride. Perhaps she enjoyed riding bikes in the morning and had done so often as a young adult. Fortunately, because Hilda's guests were not quite sure what to make of her story, they decided not to argue.

"Maybe you will be able to come along next time!" Hilda happily told her guests.

Hilda's guests did not get an actual answer about what she had done that day. They did, however, receive a very colorful story that had played out in Hilda's mind. And the situation ended positively because Hilda's guests agreed with her story. It is important to agree with a person who has dementia, even if the story she is telling is completely fabricated.

QUIZZING ABOUT FAMILY

Along the same vein, quizzing people with dementia about their family members, friends, or other visitors is also a poor decision. The grandchildren in Eleanor's story probably believed they were doing their grandmother a favor by trying to help her remember them. What they did not realize, however, is that many people with dementia live in a different world than we do, possibly in a time completely different from the actual year and month.

For example, although a man with dementia may recognize his wife, he may have a difficult time recognizing his adult children. Although this seems odd, it actually makes complete sense. His wife was already an adult when he married her. He may remember his kids, however, as toddlers or preteens. A 50-year-old woman walking in the door and calling him "Dad" might greatly confuse him. "Dad?" he may think to himself. "My daughter is 13 years old! Who is this lady?"

TIPS TO AVOID QUIZZING

The best way to approach a person with dementia, especially if you aren't sure if she will remember you, is to be calm, positive, and greet her by her first name. "Hi Joan, how are you feeling today?" you may ask. This lets Joan know that you are speaking to her and not to someone else in the room. It also gives her a sense that you are interested in her, and she will be more likely to engage positively with you. It is not uncommon to hear people with dementia say, "How did you know my name!" to a family or staff member at a dementia care community. People are always happy to be addressed personally, and they feel good that someone knows them.

This also means that staff members at care communities should not refer to residents as Honey, Sweetie, Grandma, Baby, or other terms of endearment. Half the time, residents do not realize who the staff members are even speaking to. "Grandma?" a resident may think. "I'm 25 years old! Who does this lady think she's talking to?"

Interestingly, people respond best to what they were called as children. If Joan is your mother, she may not understand when you call her "Mom," but she knows her first name. An interesting note: Women typically recognize their maiden names over their married ones because they were called "Mrs." only during the latter part of their lives. For example, if your mother's married name is Smith but her maiden name was Johnson, she may only answer to "Ms. Johnson."

Note that if your mother always remembers you, it's appropriate and expected to call her "Mom" or whatever term she responds to best. It is possible for even people with later stages of dementia to recognize close relatives and friends. It really depends on the individual. A time may come in the future, however, when your mother is not able to place you in context, and this is when you will want to start using her first name. This will eliminate any confusion and prevent her from saying, "Mom? Who are you calling Mom? Who are you?" This can be hurtful to both the person with dementia and you, the caregiver.

One of the best things to do is to talk to those with dementia about things you know they remember. Focus on past events, especially things they did as children or young adults. If your family member or friend grew up on a farm and has fond memories of helping his father feed the chickens, talk about chickens. If he loved going to the beach with the family, ask about the beach. It's best to avoid asking about the present unless you know that he'll be able to talk about it confidently. A person with dementia can find it very confusing and painful to try and remember something that happened only a few hours—or minutes—before.

If the present does come up, agree with his perception of reality. "We went biking through the mountains today!" is a good chance for you to agree and talk more about biking. "Did you have fun?" you could ask. The informative and detailed answers you receive may delight and surprise you.

Judy was ecstatic as I appeared at her door. "Guess who was here today to visit me?" she asked.

"I don't know. Who was here?" I said, smiling, unsure of the answer I would receive.

"Him!" She pointed to the television, where the president was speaking at a podium. "He was here visiting me," Judy explained happily.

Obviously, the president had not been to Judy's house that morning. Instead of arguing, however, I asked her about this experience. "Was he nice?" I asked.

"Oh, yes! We talked about politics, but I told him I didn't really like them."

"That sounds really interesting. What else did you talk about?"

"He asked about all the photos I have on the wall here," she said. "He wanted to buy them from me, but I told him that they have to stay at my house."

The president had never been to Judy's house, but the story she created was interesting and fun. She truly believed the president had visited her house. I was able to engage Judy on her level, and we had a great moment that day.

If you want to find something out about your family member or friend's care, it is best to ask the staff instead of relying on someone with dementia for accurate information. For example, your aunt with dementia may or may not be able to tell you if she took a shower, ate lunch, or had her hair done. Although she may have had a calming shower, a delicious lunch, and a great time having her perm set, she may not remember. Instead of trying to sort through her memories, talk to the staff about what she has or hasn't done that day. This will keep you from quizzing her, and you'll receive true information.

Sometimes, family members will believe what their loved ones with dementia say and then get angry at staff members at their care community.

"Mom told me that she never ate dinner last night," Bill snapped at me. "She said everyone ignored her, and she never got fed!"

"She did come out for dinner," I replied, shaking my head. "She sat at her normal table and even seemed to enjoy conversing with her friends."

"Well, she doesn't remember that," Bill said. "How do I know it happened?"

People with dementia are typically unable to recall recent events due to their damaged short-term memories. When they go searching for information, such as recalling if they ate dinner the night before, the information is not there. They cannot recall if they ate dinner, but since they do not feel full presently, they assume they did not actually eat.

Knowing that people with dementia confuse information easily, the best way to connect with them is to avoid quizzing. Instead, ask about the past, and when hearing a story from the present, embrace and accept that tale as the truth.

9

Become a Dementia Detective

Your parent, partner, child, or friend with dementia will, at some point, exhibit some odd behavioral symptoms. Perhaps you've already noticed a few bizarre changes. Maybe your partner with dementia no longer wants to take a shower. Maybe he has started urinating in your houseplants. Perhaps he has even begun hiding or hoarding items. No matter the behavior, there is always a cause—and if you are patient enough, you can probably find a solution. This is what it means to be a dementia detective: showing patience, hunting for clues, and eventually solving your family member or friend's behavioral problem.

The greatest thing about becoming a dementia detective is that it takes no previous experience. You only need two things: patience and a deep understanding of your friend or family member's needs. Recognize, however, that becoming a behavioral detective takes some practice. No one is good at it immediately, although people who have a good handle on psychology and human behavior will probably find early success. Typically, even your parent, partner, or friend's doctors will not be able to solve his behavioral problems—and many may suggest medication instead. But often, medications beget even more issues. Although they are sometimes necessary and perhaps even a good addition to problem behaviors, medications typically cannot solve an underlying issue based on something environmental. Since most doctors will not and cannot take the time to understand your family member's behaviors, the detective work is up to you.

BEHAVIORAL PROBLEMS

A little patience and a lot of trial and error can go a long way. I encountered an interesting behavioral problem at one of the communities where I worked.

"She will sit down on couches, in a chair, wherever—but I cannot get her to sit down on the toilet!" Brittany, a resident assistant, sighed. "Susannah gets really stiff and tries to hold her pants up."

Susannah was incredibly pleasant, but she was also in a moderately advanced stage of Alzheimer's disease. She walked throughout the community during the day, picking up objects; putting them down; and using short, sweet phrases to speak. Susannah particularly loved the baby dolls and stuffed animals at the dementia care community; she would carry them in her arms, cooing gently to them.

I told Brittany to come find me when Susannah needed to use the bathroom. I was intrigued by this problem and wanted to find a solution. About an hour after we spoke, Brittany brought me to Susannah's room.

Thinking that Susannah felt uncomfortable having her pants down in front of another person, I had her hold a towel in front of her legs while I reached for her pants.

"Hmmmm, yep, that's that," she said, gripping her pants so that we could not pull them down. Believing that perhaps the issue was just related to modesty, I hoped distracting her would help. I handed Susannah her favorite baby doll and asked her to look after him for a minute. "Ohh, hello," she said, smiling at the doll. This time, she let me take her pants down to her ankles while she "watched" the baby.

Brittany and I then asked her to sit down on the toilet. Susannah stiffened like a wooden board. Clearly, her pants weren't the only issue. Brittany and I tried again to get her to sit down. We walked her out of the bathroom and brought her back. We mimed sitting, hoping she would follow suit. Nothing worked.

"Do you want to sit down?" I asked Susannah.

"Hmmm, look at this," she said, misunderstanding the question and pointing to the baby. Then she said, "There's a hole."

This statement confused me at first. A hole? I wasn't sure what she was talking about. I paused, considering my options. Then, suddenly, I realized what she meant: she was afraid of the hole in the toilet.

I grabbed a bright blue towel from the bathroom wall and laid it over the toilet seat. "Hey, Susannah, sit down here," I said gently. She turned around and looked at the seat. It no longer had a hole in the middle—just a towel.

"Oh, okay," she agreed, and sat down without hesitation.

After she sat down on the new blue seat, Brittany and I gently lifted her and quickly slid the towel out from under her bottom. It was not modesty that upset her—it was the toilet itself. She was afraid of falling into the toilet bowl.

I taught this method to the rest of the care staff, who then had no more issues getting Susannah to use the bathroom.

Susannah's story provides a great example of how to put dementia detective skills to work. Although it can take some time, trial and error is the best way to solve a dementia-related problem. Once the problem is clear, it's much easier to solve.

PROBLEM-SOLVING TIPS

Fear, anxiety, pain, or another unmet basic human need motivates most dementia-related behaviors. Many people with dementia, unable to express their feelings any other way, will become combative or aggressive when hungry, tired, or in pain. In order to figure out how to solve a problem, we must know the source.

Keeping a journal is an effective way to start problem solving troubling behavior. Chart the time of day the behavior occurs. Does Aunt Margaret only start yelling for her mother around 3:00 p.m. each day? What time does Grandmom start looking for the door to leave? Determine if a pattern exists with regard to the time of day. Does it happen every day or only every once in a while? Also, look at what precedes the behavior and add that to the chart. For example, if Dad only becomes agitated after family gatherings, maybe he dislikes large crowds. What does the person with dementia say about the behavior, if he can speak?

Look for signs of discomfort or pain. When a person without dementia is in pain, he can usually explain what is happening. Even the highest-functioning people with dementia, however, seem to struggle with explaining discomfort. Keep in mind that often, a trip to the doctor is the only sure way to diagnose a physical problem. For many people with dementia, urinary tract infections (UTIs) are a common cause of behavioral change, anxiety, pain, and increased confusion. In senior-living communities in particular, UTIs are very common but also very treatable. A UTI could be the culprit for a problem behavior.

If pain is ruled out and the problem behavior still occurs, it's important to look at the person's past experiences and compare them with what is in the journal. For example, if a loved one refuses to sleep through the night and insists on napping throughout the day, look back at his history. Did this person ever work a third shift earlier in life? Even if he hasn't worked the third shift in decades, this information is still very important. It could easily explain the new, bizarre sleeping patterns: he believes that work starts at 11:00 p.m.

Rob was convinced that snakes bit his toes at night while he slept. "I can't sleep in there anymore!" he cried out. "The snakes are in my covers, and they are nipping at my toes. I can feel them slithering in my bed while I'm trying to sleep!"

Rob had dementia with Lewy bodies, which meant he tended to hallucinate. His current hallucination, the snakes, were preventing him from sleeping. His family didn't know what to do. At first, they argued with him. "Dad, look," his daughter, Angela, said. She pulled back the covers on his bed and switched on the light. "See? There aren't any snakes in here," she said, trying to comfort him. "It's just your imagination! Go back to sleep."

This only frustrated Rob further: he was sure there were snakes in his bed, and now his family just thought he was crazy. Rob's dementia prevented him from understanding that the snakes were not real, but fortunately, he was able to verbally communicate the problem: he was afraid.

Eventually, his daughter decided to embrace his reality and try to find a solution that would suit Rob's needs. The family filled an empty spray bottle with water and added lavender, a calming scent. "Here, Dad," Angela offered, handing him the bottle. "This should take care of your problem. This spray bottle is full of snake repellent. Anytime you see or feel a snake, just spray the bed. It should start to work immediately!"

Rob was able to use his "snake repellent" to take care of his hallucination. Because his family embraced his reality and dealt effectively with his fear, Rob was finally able to sleep through the night. Eventually, Rob was able to stop using it entirely. As time went on, his fear, and his snake hallucination, faded.

Rob's family was fortunate because he was able to tell them about his problem. For people who cannot speak, problem solving can be much more challenging. Following a few simple tactics, however, can save caregivers a lot of time and energy.

PRESSING ON

Above all else, problem solving means trial and error. Based on the journal, the pain assessment, and knowledge of a person's past experiences, you can learn a lot. Although a number of attempts may fail before something works, it is important to keep hunting. It's important to note, also, that what worked one day may not work another day. For example, what did not work on Tuesday may actually end up working on Wednesday. What worked on Thursday may not work again on Monday. Although this can be frustrating, it's about human behavior—people change their minds and their moods all the time. That is what makes dementia care so difficult.

And of course, try not to resent a person with dementia for behaving strangely at times. Remember that it is not the person's fault and press on. As a dementia detective, it is imperative to keep digging, keep discovering, and keep attempting new solutions.

10

Car Keys, Cell Phones, and Wallets

Many caregivers struggle with the idea that they must, at some point, begin taking things away from their parent, partner, child, or friend with dementia. When is it time to take away a person's car keys? What about the person's cell phone? And, especially as an even more tech-savvy future awaits us, what about the Internet? Even if a person with dementia moves into a dementia care community, these questions remain important to tackle.

Most people have a list of objects they grab before leaving the house. For many, the list is the same. Wallet or purse? Check. Car keys? Yes. Cell phone? Check. The minute any of these items go missing, most people begin to panic. Someone with dementia feels the same anxiety. Caregivers need to decide when the time is right to take important items from a family member with dementia, or at least prevent the person from using the item, especially a set of car keys.

THE WALLET

Ed began checking his pockets. "Where is my wallet?" he asked himself. Ed, at 83 years old, lived in a dementia care community. For as long as he could remember, he had carried a wallet in his back pocket. Now it was nowhere to be found. As the minutes ticked by, Ed became more and more upset. "Which one of you stole my wallet!" he shouted, pointing to a group of staff members.

The problem was that Ed hadn't carried a wallet in years. His family had taken the wallet so that he would not lose it or use any money or credit cards. Ed could not remember this, however. His agitation finally subsided, only to pick back up again hours later at dinner when he reached into his pocket in an attempt to pay for his meal.

Ed's family likely did him a disservice by removing his wallet. They felt it was the only way to keep him from losing it or mishandling money, but Ed didn't understand that. Instead, he blamed other people for stealing the wallet.

A number of ideas can prevent a person with dementia from panicking about his wallet. The first and easiest option is to allow the person to keep a wallet, but buy a few of them (cheaply, if possible). Put the wallets around the person's room and in a few pockets, purses, or drawers. Neither the original nor the replacement wallets should contain anything valuable, however, or be valuable themselves.

For people using walkers or wheelchairs, purchasing a basket or even a walker with a seat is another great option. Wallets or purses can fit into these compartments and stay with the person wherever he or she goes. It is probably still wise to offer a few replacements, but most people with gait impairments take their walking aids with them everywhere. Items stored in these aids are less likely to go missing.

For people in the earlier stages of dementia, hang a hook or put a basket in their room to store the wallet or purse. This may help someone easily find an item. Labeling a drawer or nook in a person's room is also a good idea. Staff members in dementia care communities will find objects and put them back where they came from as long as they know where they go.

Cancel credit or debit cards before placing them into a wallet. In fact, inactive credit cards are a great way to provide a sense of comfort and normalcy to a person with dementia. Be sure there is no way for the person to contact the credit card company and get a new card. Alert the staff at the dementia care community that the cards are inactive, so they don't worry about them getting lost.

Betty had a tendency to call the police any chance she got. Because her family allowed her to keep a phone in her room at her dementia care community, Betty called the police often. Dialing 9-1-1 was a lot easier than calling a family member, particularly because Betty had to dial out of the community first to reach anyone.

This time, Betty called the police about her credit cards. "My family stole my credit cards," she complained to the police. "I need you guys to go to their house and get me the cards!" Betty's family had removed her credit cards because they knew she would try to use or misplace them.

"Can you please give Betty her cards back but just cancel them ahead of time?" I asked her family. "She won't stop calling the police!"

The police had to come every time they were called. Her family ended up having to pay the bill that the city charged for sending them over to review Betty's nonsensical phone calls.

Many people also carry cash with them on a regular basis. Families often struggle with this because people with dementia cannot manage money effectively. Allowing a person with dementia to have a few dollars in a wallet or purse is usually acceptable, as long as everyone recognizes that such money disappears often and will be impossible to find later. For people in later stages of dementia, play money should also work. A party store is a great place to purchase fake dollar bills. In dementia care communities, in particular, residents are often concerned about paying for their meals. They don't want to feel as though someone is serving them for free and often try to "leave a tip" or ask for the check. Providing fake money or canceled credit cards is a perfect way to give a person with dementia some sense of autonomy.

Be sure to label everything. When items go missing, especially in dementia care communities, staff members can have difficulty figuring out what belongs to whom. Writing a name in a person's wallet will increase the chances that the wallet will get back to its rightful owner.

THE CAR KEYS

When is it time to take away a parent, partner, or sibling with dementia's car keys? This is a very common and complex question. When the person begins to get lost, drive dangerously, ignore road signs, or seem confused about how to start or stop a vehicle, it is absolutely time for that person to stop driving. Of course, preventing a person from driving is much more challenging than noticing he shouldn't be driving in the first place.

Although some people with dementia may actually agree to stop driving, many will put up a fight. An adult child or a spouse saying, "You cannot drive any longer" likely will not convince them. Most people do not want to be told to stop driving, especially when they have been driving for decades. For many caregivers, getting another party involved is the best way to stop someone with dementia from operating a vehicle.

One popular technique to prevent a person from driving is to involve a doctor. Tell the doctor ahead of time that your family member should probably not be driving any longer, and the doctor can help make the official call. Hearing the bad news from a doctor will be a lot easier than hearing it from you, the caregiver. This will also prevent your loved one from taking out his anger on you.

Another option is to contact your local fire or police department. Many local agencies have programs that help stop people with dementia from driving. An officer can pull your family member or friend over and suggest a driving test. Although he is going to be angry, it's not your fault. He won't blame you and will instead feel as though a third party is responsible for the change. The most important thing is that your family member or friend is safe and no longer behind the wheel of a vehicle.

Even though a person with dementia can no longer drive,

typically, the battle is not over. Many people with dementia forget they do not have the ability to drive and will go in search of the car or the keys to the car.

It was getting dark outside, and Lisa felt like it was time to leave. She believed she was staying in a hotel, even though she was really just sitting in the living room of the house she had lived in for 50 years. Lisa looked at her watch. "Eight o' clock?" she asked, mystified. "Where did the time go? It's getting late, and we should be going."

Lisa reached over to the side table to look for her car keys. "Where are my keys now?" she asked.

"Oh, Lisa," her caregiver offered. "I forgot to tell you that I took your car to the shop today. Something was wrong with the motor, and I wanted to make sure that we got it fixed for you." This wasn't true, of course, because the car was sitting in the driveway.

"Oh, really?" Lisa asked. "Well, thank you for getting that fixed. I guess we can just stay here another night until it's ready to go."

Different techniques will work for different people. The approach that Lisa's caregiver used will not work for everyone. If your mother asks about her car keys, perhaps you can suggest they got lost somewhere in the house. Maybe the car has a flat tire. Perhaps someone is borrowing the vehicle for the afternoon. No matter what, recall that embracing the reality of the person with dementia is key and that reorientation is never the answer. "Mom, you can't drive anymore, remember?" is a statement that starts a fight—not ends one.

Like the wallet scenario, providing your mother with a deactivated car key may help. As long as the car key does not actually work, it may reassure her to feel as though she has the key to the car in hand. Consider keeping a few old car keys lying around in case the original gets lost.

THE CELL PHONE

Caregivers often wonder if they should provide their family members who have dementia with a phone. Typically, the answer is no: It is a bad idea for a person with moderate to advanced dementia to have a phone. Although some people with dementia can use a phone appropriately, most do not understand times of day and will call loved ones at odd hours. Betty's story earlier in this chapter illustrates one of the dangers of allowing a person with dementia to have a phone. Because she couldn't understand the world around her, Betty phoned the police whenever she was upset or anxious.

Phones made specifically for people with dementia are available online. These corded phones lack a keypad, so there are no numbers to push. Family members can call in, and if the person with dementia is in the room, she can pick up the phone and talk. Because these phones do not have dialing-out options, family members don't have to contend with frequent calls from loved ones at inappropriate hours. These types of phones will also prevent people with dementia from ordering expensive items from television shopping channels, phoning the police, or placing calls to their bank or credit-card companies.

The increase in cell-phone usage is likely to increase the problems for people with dementia. People in later stages of dementia may regularly misplace their phones. On top of this, many people with dementia will not understand how to use a phone as their dementia progresses. A land-line phone that doesn't allow a person to dial out is a good option in this case. Caregivers may also want to look into keeping a few broken cell phones on hand. If the phone does not have a SIM card or a battery, there is likely no harm in a person with dementia carrying a cell phone around. You can also disable the phone so that its owner cannot call out, by terminating the contract with the service provider. There is no doubt that in the near future people with dementia are going to spend significant amounts of time searching for missing cell phones.

INTERNET USAGE

This is new ground for dementia caregiving. Probably one of the best things that a caregiver can do is limit their family member or friend's access to the Internet. Most computers or Internet service providers offer website safeguards, typically used to prevent children from viewing certain pages. Caregivers may deem it necessary to place certain safeguards on e-mail or other sites to prevent their family members from doing any social harm to themselves in the early stages of dementia. Also, many opportunities exist for con artists to trick people with dementia using spam e-mails or fake advertisements. It's important to keep your loved one from engaging in scams on the web.

Bennett had been sending his family a lot of bizarre e-mails. His daughter wasn't sure what he was talking about half the time, and she grew concerned when he began posting odd statuses on his newly acquired Facebook page. E-mails came in at midnight, 3:00 a.m., and 6:00 a.m. When she asked him about it, Bennett just explained that he was afraid of missing important messages and stayed up waiting for them to come in.

Although this is not currently a problem for most people with dementia, as time goes on more and more people will have dementia-related trouble with social media outlets on the web. The people now using the Internet on a regular basis will likely want to continue, even if they have dementia. It is likely that a person with dementia will have trouble using social media, surfing the web, and using e-mail. These problems will probably be more evident in the early stages of dementia because people in later stages will likely stop using the Internet altogether.

HANDLING IT WITH GRACE

Caregivers have a hard job, especially when it entails taking things away from their parent, partner, child, or friend with dementia. Be it a cell phone, car keys, the Internet, or a wallet, there are ways to handle the change with grace and empathy. People with dementia are still people—and they do not want to be stripped of things that are part of their daily routine. It is important that, as caregivers, we respect their desire for autonomy while finding ways to keep them happy and safe.

PART III

LIVING IN A DEMENTIA CARE COMMUNITY

11

The Importance of Meaningful Activities

I walked through the community's doors and scanned the area around me. Six residents sat asleep in front of the television. The wall in front of me was decorated like a child's bedroom, with stickers, block lettering, and bright colors. "Welcome!!!" the wall screamed in big letters. Down the hall sat a long row of chairs in which a number of residents were positioned. Most were asleep, but some stared off into the distance. Down another hall, a scream rang out. A woman was wheeling herself down the hallway in her wheelchair and crying for her parents. The staff members didn't seem to notice.

Besides the roar of the television blasting rap music from MTV, no other music sounded in the hallway. A resident wandered past me, and I smiled and offered my hand. She took it and looked up at me, pleased at the attention. Staff members rushed nearby and seemed preoccupied with their own agendas. The walls were marked with boilerplate, framed images—some of flowers, some of buildings, others of people playing in the ocean. The photographs were randomly arranged, seemingly without purpose.

No evidence of activities existed at this community: no boxes of items for residents to tinker with, no life-skills stations, no baby dolls, no music, nothing.

A place like this one is not a place where residents enjoy life—it is a place where people go to pass away slowly. I wish that I could say this describes one dementia care community in particular, but it does not; very sadly, it describes many dementia care communities. The goal at any community should be to create a world where the residents are happy, engaged, and excited about life.

SEARCHING FOR THE RIGHT COMMUNITY

When looking for a community for your family member or friend, thorough research is imperative. You should attempt to find one that best matches your loved one's needs as well as offers numerous and varying activities and programs every day. Even though medical care is extremely important in a care community, it's not the only thing keeping residents healthy. Healthy residents are well cared for in both body and soul. They are not necessarily happy even in a place with wonderful medical care, hygiene, and meals if activities fall by the wayside. Residents experience more agitation, anxiety, and depression when they are not actively engaged—and this takes a toll on them physically. When a community fails to provide meaningful activities, outings, and entertainment, residents take more medication, sundown more, and sleep constantly. A place that offers activities provides—without a doubt—a better life for its residents.

I walked through the doors into the dementia care community and immediately heard music playing from the CD player across the hall. Elvis Presley crooned, and a resident sat on the couch nearby, tapping his foot and nodding his head in time to the beat. Six residents sat in chairs in an activity space, all occupied. Two residents worked together folding and matching baby socks while two more put a puzzle together. Another resident was matching cards, and still another sat nearby, seeming to oversee the whole operation. A staff member helped the two women arranging socks, offering one after another. "How about this one? Does this match anything?" she asked.

The television in the middle of the wall played an old movie, loud enough for residents to hear. Three residents sat near it, engaged in the movie. I walked down the hallway and passed a life-skills station set up with baby clothing and a crib. A baby doll lay in the crib, and a resident sat nearby in the rocking chair, cradling another doll while rocking back and forth. She smiled to herself and sang quietly to the doll. A resident walked past me, pushing a stuffed dog on his walker. "What a great-looking dog you have!" I said to him.

"He's a good puppy most of the time," the man smiled back.

In another room, the activity director was conducting a painting class. Residents worked diligently on their canvases, and their previous pieces covered the wall. The colors and themes were inviting and warm. Everywhere, staff seemed relaxed. Although it could be a stressful environment at times, the entire community had the air of a place where people truly enjoyed life.

Maybe this type of community seems like a fantasy but it exists, and I have worked in communities like this one. I have spent countless hours, days, weeks, and months building communities like this one. The most important measure of any dementia care community, truly, is how it feels upon first walking through its doors. Trust your first impressions and reactions. Are residents engaged? Are they involved in activities, or are they assembled in front of a television set? Is appropriate music playing or is the music inappropriate for the residents? Or is the place silent? Are people smiling, laughing, and talking to one another or asleep? How does the staff act when you come in the door? Do they greet you, or do they seem to ignore you? The answers to these questions can tell you a lot about a community.

Baby dolls, stuffed animals, music, and more all create a positive, engaging environment in dementia care. Residents also need to be active in programs throughout the day. The most successful communities involve both resident-care associates and the activity director in making sure that residents have something to do. Resident-care associates run smaller programs with residents who may be lower functioning, while the activity director engages residents who have higher-functioning needs. This way, the majority of residents take part in activities that meet their level of need. No one becomes frustrated because their activities are too difficult or bored because their activities are too simple.

It's not uncommon to hear family members say things like "Mom can't do much of anything anymore. She mostly likes to sit around and watch TV." While this may be true, it is up to a good activity director to find something the resident would enjoy doing.

EXAMPLES OF ACTIVITIES

People who have dementia may enjoy some of the following activities. The amount and type of activity needed will vary depending on a person's type and level of dementia. Although some activities, like sorting socks, will work well for a person in later-stage dementia, the same activity may bore someone in an earlier stage.

Sorting Socks

Generally, sorting socks is a fantastic activity for people with dementia. Although laundry is typically not a favorite chore for most people, asking those with dementia to "help" with sock sorting can provide them with a wonderful opportunity. Most people want to help others, and as the disease progresses, people with dementia rarely get asked to assist with tasks any longer. A simple "Can you help me fold and match these socks?" is likely to get a positive response from almost any resident who wants something to do.

Folding Towels

Folding towels is the same type of activity as matching socks. Residents typically enjoy the activity because it feels useful—most people have folded towels often in their lives. It feels like a necessary, important task to keep a household running. This type of activity can bring back memories of homemaking and raising children.

Matching Items

Some people enjoy strategy and thinking games, so matching cards or pictures is good for residents who can no longer complete more challenging brain games. An easy way to set up this type of activity is to lay colorful cards or pictures on a table and ask for "help" sorting through all of them. This can also work with holiday cards.

Matching Lids to Jars

Sorting through Tupperware isn't usually fun, but it gives people with dementia the opportunity to "help" another person and a welcome chance to do something useful. A mismatch of jars, containers, and lids can provide a person with dementia a chance to sort and match the items.

Building Blocks

More creative people, especially men who spent years building or working with their hands, may appreciate the opportunity to build or create things. It is important that the blocks or pieces used for building are not childish or too colorful. When given the chance to create something, it's amazing to see what people with dementia can come up with.

Lacing and Tracing Kits

Sewing, especially threading a tiny needle, can present a huge challenge to a person with poor eyesight or arthritic hands. A "lace and trace" kit can be found online or in many stores' game sections. These kits usually include a few different shapes with holes around the perimeter. The user threads a colorful string in and out of these holes, moving around the shape. The motion is similar to sewing, but it is much easier to see and to hold.

Singing

Those with dementia can often recall lyrics and melodies to favorite songs. It is amazing to see this in action. Even when it seems like other memories are gone, the ability to sing along to an old tune remains. For many people in dementia care communities, perhaps the best part of any day is when an entertainer comes in to sing or play music. Pianists, singers, guitar players, accordion players, and dancers are sure to please at dementia care communities.

Fill in the Blank

Like music, fill-in-the-blank cards can work wonders for people with dementia. For example, starting an old lyric like "I found my thrill . . ." gives someone time to fill in the rest of the sentence. "On Blueberry Hill!" he may say. Games that allow people with dementia to think back to old sayings, phrases, and lyrics are usually very successful and popular.

Completing Puzzles

Not everyone enjoys putting a puzzle together, but many people with dementia relish the ability to complete something, especially when they feel as though they have done it themselves. Puzzles for people with dementia should have large, easy-to-see pieces and fewer than 50 parts that fit together. Anything bigger becomes overwhelming and typically leads to frustration and anger.

Painting

A canvas and some pots of paint give people who have dementia one of the most creative and entertaining things to do. "Paint whatever you like" is a great opener for this type of activity. It's really interesting to see what a person will create when given the opportunity. If this activity becomes too difficult, something simpler, like painting the sides and roof of a premade wooden birdhouse, may work best. A few simple instructions are better than many instructions. An invitation such as "Can you help me paint this?" receives a positive response from most adults with dementia.

Decorating

Some people with dementia enjoy decorating for holidays.

At one of my dementia care communities, my residents loved setting up for holiday events. One woman in particular spent about an hour meticulously decorating one of our Christmas trees. Clearly, she had done that in her own home and welcomed the chance to do it again. Realize that you may need to modify the activity slightly so that the person with dementia can feel successful. In the example of the tree decor, I handed items to my resident, and she put them on the tree. She was in charge of everything else, but because I handed her one ornament at a time, she was able to focus and avoid getting distracted or frustrated.

Doing What They Have Always Loved

"When is payroll due?" James asked, walking into my office.

"What?" I asked, surprised by the question. I remembered, suddenly, that James had been an accountant his whole life. The well-dressed man was 100 years old, but he still believed that he had to go to work each and every day. "Uh, it's due today. Let me get you the paperwork," I offered. "Give me a few minutes."

James nodded and left. I threw together a spreadsheet with different numbers and printed it out. I hoped he would be able to add and subtract the numbers on the spreadsheet. I also found a pencil and a calculator and carried all of these to James. He took the materials and went toward his room. "I'm going to take these back to my office," he said, walking away.

About an hour later, James emerged from his "office." "I finished payroll," he said, smiling, as he offered me the worksheet and pencil.

James didn't want to fold socks or listen to music. He wanted to do what he had always done—he wanted to go to work. Working made James feel useful, smart, and successful. Allowing James to do something he felt was necessary and important was just as good—and perhaps even better—than any other activity he could have done.

Even though James did not really do payroll, I still gave him a challenge. Although you may need to adapt your parent, partner, child, or friend's old career into something more manageable for him when he has dementia, he can still feel successful doing something he has always done.

BRINGING JOY

There is no one-size-fits-all activity for every person with dementia. But letting a person with dementia sit in front of the television all day or sleep doesn't make for a fulfilling, happy life. When caregivers say things like "Mom doesn't want to do anything anymore" or "My husband can't do much—he just likes to sit and watch movies all day" they are missing a great opportunity to provide their family member or partner with a feeling of satisfaction and worth.

Meaningful activities will not cure people who have cognitive loss, but the joy and the comfort they bring can completely change the way a person with dementia interacts with the world. Adults with dementia who have nothing to do are more irritable, more depressed, and more anxious. We all, as humans, want to feel useful and successful—and that does not stop just because we get dementia.

12

Baby Dolls, Artificial Pets, and the Importance of Environment

I was happily giving a tour of my dementia care community to a prospective family. I always enjoyed providing tours because I felt quite proud of what we had accomplished at the community. I liked to show off our life-skills stations: the baby doll area where residents would cuddle dolls, the desk and workspace for residents who felt as though they had to go to work, and even the dress-up area that looked like a woman's bedroom.

As I walked the family through our baby station, I pointed to the dolls. "Our residents really love this space," I explained, smiling. "They enjoy singing to the babies and rocking them back and forth in this rocking chair. Many take the babies back to their rooms. As you can see, we treat the babies as though they are real, because many of our residents believe they are." Turning to face the family, I saw the adult son shake his head.

"What a sad disease," he said angrily.

I was slightly stunned and didn't know how to respond. "But doesn't he see how wonderful this baby station is?" I thought to myself. It took me a moment to realize that many people who don't understand dementia could find this environment scary and bizarre.

We continued the tour, but my positive attitude was shaken. I was not sure what else to point out about the community, and I felt like I must have sounded naïve, speaking so excitedly about baby dolls. I had no easy way to explain to this man why baby dolls made my residents so happy. He probably thought we should have been trying to bring the residents back to our reality instead of embracing the world in which they lived.

Environment is an incredibly important part of dementia care. People with dementia need—and deserve—to live in an environment that provides them with comfort, security, and happiness. That's why the best dementia care communities have spaces like the one mentioned above. Life-skills stations, or places where residents can interact with relatable and comforting items, are integral parts of good care communities. Even when a person lives at home, there are still opportunities to create meaningful, pleasant spaces to ease anxiety.

BABY DOLLS

Much of a positive dementia care environment goes back to embracing the reality of the person with dementia. A caregiver who provides a baby doll to someone with dementia, for example, is embracing that person's reality. Many people with dementia believe that baby dolls are real babies, and the caregiver is accepting that fact. Caregivers commonly ask, "Why does my loved one believe that a fake baby is real?" The answer lies in the way that dementia changes the brain. As the brain degrades, so does a person's ability to perceive, understand, and comprehend. Even if a baby doll does not cry, breathe, urinate, or require food, a person with dementia is unable to understand that the baby is not real. If it looks and feels real enough, it becomes real for the person with dementia. As long as caregivers play along and treat the baby doll the same way they would treat a live baby, those with dementia may not be able to tell the difference.

Although it was typically women who found the baby dolls fascinating, John had also come to love the infants. "Are you sleepy?

Just go ahead and go to sleep," he said to the doll, rocking it softly. "Shhhh."

It was a beautiful sight to see. John enjoyed rocking and cradling the babies. His children said he had been a great father, particularly when they were very young. He loved caring for children, and the baby dolls gave him a way to keep doing that.

"Hey, John, can you watch this baby for me?" a staff member asked. "I think she needs to go down for her nap soon." Because the staff treated the dolls as though they were real, they were able to keep the story alive for John.

One morning a staff member walked in to find John cradling one of the baby dolls. He hushed the staffer. "Shh," he whispered, "I heard the baby crying."

Although these babies didn't actually cry, John's brain created a meaningful moment for him surrounding the dolls. It made sense that the baby would cry—that is what babies do, after all. And, because he thought that this baby needed his help, John felt important and useful.

Providing dolls to a person with dementia endows him with a sense of confidence and purpose. When asked to hold a baby, many people feel entrusted with a new responsibility, and people with dementia are no different. It is still important for those with dementia to feel necessary and independent. Caring for a child, real or not, is a fantastic opportunity for a person with dementia to be a caregiver again. Typically, baby dolls will also bring up memories for those with dementia. It's not uncommon to hear people reminisce about caring for their own children or what it was like growing up with their parents.

FAKE PETS

Stuffed animals—or real ones, for that matter—have a similar effect on people with dementia as babies do. Stuffed animals are particularly useful for people in later stages of dementia because they neither require care nor do they accidentally scratch or bite the delicate skin that older adults have. People who have grown up caring for animals usually love looking after a stuffed animal. Holding or cuddling a fake pet can bring immense comfort even to people who do not believe the animal is real.

"Ohh," Gertrude whispered. "Is he for me?" She reached out to take the small stuffed dog. He looked remarkably realistic, even down to the softness of his fur.

"Sure, you can have him," I said, smiling as I handed her the stuffed animal.

Gertrude loved dogs. I knew she had owned a number of dogs in her life, and she was always excited when therapy dogs came in to visit with the residents. Recalling this, I hoped she would have the same reaction if handed a stuffed dog—and did she ever. Gertrude embraced the dog gently, holding him to her chest. "Oh, you are the sweetest thing," she whispered, closing her eyes and petting the dog's fur. "I will take the best care of you."

Whenever Gertrude became upset or anxious, we brought her the stuffed dog. Her reaction was the same every time: surprise, delight, and pure happiness. She thought we were entrusting her with the dog's care—and this meant a lot to her. She also believed the dog was real, and it gave her a chance to have a pet again. Just because Gertrude's dog was a stuffed toy did not mean that it did not have the same effect as a real dog.

Some dementia care communities have pet stations, just as they have baby-skills stations. For ones that do not, caregivers are welcome to provide a stuffed animal to their family member or friend. As long as these pets are labeled, they are unlikely to go missing, at least permanently. Some care communities also allow real pets to live with their owners. Typically, in the later stages of dementia, this becomes a problem. People with dementia are often unable to get themselves to the bathroom, let alone care for a pet's waste. Sometimes, it is best to have a family member care for the owner's pet when the owner moves into a care community. Caregivers can then give their loved one a similarly sized stuffed animal, if they think it will comfort the person. In many cases, it does.

MUSIC

Listening to music is an important part of many people's lives. For those with dementia, hearing music can have an extremely positive effect on behavior. They often remember lyrics or tunes long after other memories have faded.

"I found my thrill on Blueberry Hill, on Blueberry Hill, where I found you," the residents sang in unison. Even if the lyrics had not been on the television screen, they would have known the song. Music and lyrics have a profound effect on most people in the world. For our residents with dementia, this effect was perhaps even stronger. Where other memories had faded, the lyrics and tunes of songs had stayed. In order to keep the positive energy flowing throughout the community, we installed CD players in most common areas. Pleasant, upbeat music played on repeat all day, every day.

Playing music in common areas for residents or even providing them with personal music players is a great way to keep them happy. Music has an impact on mood, and for people with dementia, keeping the mood pleasant and comfortable is essential. In dining areas, communities can play music during meals, just as restaurants normally do. It's best if the music does not have lyrics, because some residents will get caught up singing and forget to eat. Keeping the mood positive is an important step in getting residents to enjoy mealtimes and hopefully, eat more.

LIGHTING

Changes in lighting strongly affect people with dementia. Dark rooms with no windows are usually troublesome. A dark room implies that it is nighttime, making people sleepy. Darkness also creates a fall hazard because aging adults often have impaired vision.

A well-lit room with windows that is painted in warm colors does wonders for people with dementia. This is important to keep in mind not only when visiting dementia care communities but also for people with dementia living at home. Lighting and room color affect everything from sleeping to eating. People in well-lit spaces are more likely to stay awake instead of nodding off to sleep throughout the day.

FLOORING AND PATTERNS

Just as people with dementia perceive baby dolls to be real, their perception of patterns and flooring can become distorted. Chairs, carpets, or tablecloths with patterns tend to confuse those with dementia. For example, a carpet with a leaf pattern may encourage residents to bend down and attempt to pick up the leaves. A tablecloth with zigzag lines and bright colors may cause a person with dementia to spend time playing with the cloth instead of focusing on a plate of food. Even carpets with thick lines, or dark-colored rugs, can cause difficulties.

The different colors in the carpet perplexed Joan. Because a thick, dark green line went across the light green carpet, it looked to Joan as though there was a hole in the floor. Joan's dementia disturbed her spatial and depth perception.

Every time she walked by the line, she stepped over it. Usually, she would stop, pick up her cane, and put it on the other side of the line. Joan would then gingerly step over the line. Afraid that others might fall through the floor, she would often stand by the spot, warning residents of what she perceived to be a dangerous situation.

Similarly, floor rugs not only cause falls but can cause confusion when dark in color. Like Joan, many people with dementia have difficulty discriminating between a hole in the floor and a dark-colored piece of fabric. Using patternless fabrics and flooring are important in dementia care.

THE REWARD

Building a positive environment for a person with dementia takes some creativity, but it doesn't require a lot of resources. For example, if you know that your mother with dementia loves looking after children, she may enjoy a baby doll. Buying a realistic-looking baby doll and a couple of different outfits does not have to be expensive or time consuming. Even if your loved one lives in a care community with no baby station, there is no reason you cannot suggest that the community create a space for a crib. If that isn't possible, you could give your loved one a doll to carry with her and hold in her lap. Perhaps providing him with a CD or MP3 player would allow him to enjoy his favorite music. Or, choosing attractive pillows for your loved one's bed might encourage her to sleep there. A number of options are available to create a welcoming environment where a person with dementia can thrive.

Creating life-skills stations and modifying a person's environment can be enjoyable, especially when your efforts pay off. When you find that your mother enjoys her dolls, is less agitated, and generally seems happier, any time or money spent pays off tenfold. A person with dementia requires a positive, engaging environment to live a happy, fulfilling life. People with dementia may have a disease, but their lives don't have to end the minute they receive the diagnosis.

13

A Note about Visiting

One big reason people shy away from visiting family members or friends in dementia care is because they feel uncomfortable when entering the community. Visitors aren't sure how to talk to a resident or what to talk about. They may feel awkward, anxious, or even bored. What many people do not realize, however, are the many things visitors can do when seeing a parent, partner, adult child, or friend in a dementia care community.

HOW TO PROCEED

One of the best things a visitor can do is to bring something meaningful from home. A photo album is a great way to connect with a family member or friend in dementia care. Even if the person with dementia cannot name everyone in the photos, he'll get a lot of joy out of browsing through them with you. Don't be alarmed if he confuses or misunderstands who or what is in the photo. Go along with his story. You may learn something about your parent or partner that you didn't know before.

Be sure to label anything you bring and leave with your family member or friend. Glasses, shoes, clothing, games, stuffed animals, and more go missing on a regular basis at most communities, typically because other residents pick them up and carry them around. This frustrates a lot of family members. This is the nature of dementia care, however—residents forget items, take them off, put them down, and another resident picks them up. Labeling items may help them get back to the rightful owner.

It's also a great idea to bring in a homemade baked good or meal. Perhaps your mom lives in a dementia care community but enjoyed baking pies when she lived at home. Find one of her favorite recipes and try your hand at it. Many communities have small kitchens where activity directors can bake with the residents. If your mom's community allows it, you could also bring ingredients and bake with her right there in the kitchen. You may also discover that your mom enjoys reading through old recipes. Recall that long-term memories stay with a person much longer than short-term memories. If your mom loved baking, talking about and looking at old recipes may bring up some strong, happy emotions. Note, however, that you should be aware of her diet plan and what she cannot eat.

Bring a pet into the community for a visit. Many family members with calm dogs will bring them to senior communities to visit. Seeing a beloved pet from home—or any pet for people who like them—can be an incredibly happy experience for those with dementia. Alternatively, a stuffed animal or even a baby doll will often provide the same type of positive interaction. Knowing what your family member or friend will and will not enjoy is key here.

Choose some music that your parent, partner, or sibling enjoys and bring that with you when you visit. Play it through a speaker so that you can both listen or even keep it on in the background while you talk. For most people, music is a powerful tool for bringing back memories and emotions. Songs from a person's childhood garner a particularly strong emotional reaction.

"I found my thrill, on Blueberry Hill, where I found you," all of the residents sang. Even though we played "Blueberry Hill" nearly every day, no one ever got tired of it. Our residents absolutely loved that song. When it came on over the karaoke speakers, all of the residents stopped what they were doing to sing.

Lila, in particular, loved "Blueberry Hill." Typically, it was hard to get Lila out of her room. "No, I'm too tired," she would say. "I can't come out right now." As soon as we cued up her favorite song, though, Lila would come waltzing out her door. "You're playing my song!" she would cry out. Her feet would move gracefully across the floor—so much so that she often forgot her walker inside her room.

Watching the residents sing along to particular songs was always a magical experience. Although many could not remember what they had eaten for breakfast, they remembered all of the words to their favorite songs. They would often recount far-gone memories, too. "My husband and I used to go out dancing all the time!" a resident said one time, offering a story I had never heard her mention before.

Dementia seems to affect the brain very little when it comes to music. Letting a person with dementia listen to music from a bygone era can be very rewarding. A gift for a resident in the form of a CD player or MP3 player with headphones can also work wonders, particularly for people who get agitated when there is a lot of commotion. In order to decrease the chance that a music player will get lost or go missing, it may be easiest to take the music player home after the visit.

A FAMILY AFFAIR

Planning a trip outside the community can also lead to a positive experience for both the caregiver and the resident. Enjoying a meal together at a nearby restaurant or even eating together inside the community can be a great opportunity for conversation. Even if your family member or friend with dementia cannot speak much or at all, he can still enjoy your company.

Roger didn't talk much. Although he was often pleasant and engaging, he rarely strung an entire sentence together. If anything, Roger just uttered a short phrase or two. He enjoyed being the center of attention and often "told" jokes using physical gestures and funny facial expressions.

It was Roger's birthday, and his family had planned a unique party for him. Knowing that it would be difficult to take him out for the afternoon, they brought the party to him. After checking with the community to ensure that it was acceptable, the family set up camp in one of the common areas. They brought in a cake, presents, and even decorations. Roger loved the attention, even though it was not clear if he knew exactly what was happening.

Roger's family were aware of his limitations. They understood that he would likely not know that it was his birthday, and they realized he would probably have trouble blowing out candles or opening presents. The family knew, though, that Roger loved visitors and enjoyed eating cake. They modified his birthday party to meet his needs, and everyone enjoyed the outcome.

You can choose any number of items or gifts to bring with you to the care community to connect with your friend or family member. The best thing you can bring, however, is a positive attitude. You may see, hear, or encounter some things while visiting that you didn't expect. The best way to handle such a challenging experience is to prepare yourself ahead of time.

14

Personal Preferences

A resident's personal preferences are particularly important in dementia care. Many care communities ask caregivers to fill out questionnaires about their family member or friend before that person moves into the community. Although the list of questions may seem lengthy and some of the questions may seem strange, family members help the person with dementia by answering all of the questions. Most people with dementia cannot accurately describe their likes and dislikes, so the information on a questionnaire is vitally important to their comfort and satisfaction.

After spending enough time with their residents, staff members eventually get to know them, but before that they can learn much useful information from the family questionnaire and apply it first-hand to the resident's care. For example, if the staff at a care community know before meeting your mom not to mention her ex-husband, they will not make the mistake of bringing up her marriage. If they know your dad only drinks his tea with milk and sugar, they will not have to spend days trying to figure out why he keeps spitting out his unsweetened tea at mealtimes. It's worth repeating that personal preferences play a huge role in positive dementia caregiving. Providing community staff with information about your parent, partner, or friend will enhance their ability to provide wonderful care.

"Mom loves to drink coffee in the morning," Jane explained to the staff at her mother's dementia care community. "Please make sure that she gets a cup."

The next morning, the staff prepared Evelyn's coffee and served it to her in the dining room. Evelyn had moderate to advanced dementia, but she was still able to use utensils and eat without assistance. She looked at the cup of hot coffee that morning, however, and continued to eat her breakfast. "What's wrong, Evelyn?" a staff member asked. "You don't like coffee?"

Evelyn seemed confused by the question and continued to eat. She left the table that morning without drinking any of her coffee. For the next five days, the reaction was the same. Evelyn looked at the coffee and ignored it. The staff offered her cream and sugar, hoping that would solve the problem, but she ignored this as well.

Evelyn's daughter came to visit the next weekend, and a staff member approached her regarding the coffee situation. "Your mom doesn't seem to like coffee anymore," the staff member said. "We bring her a hot cup every morning, and we even offer cream and sugar. Maybe she just doesn't enjoy coffee these days."

Jane paused and thought for a moment. "Oh, mom always had a newspaper in front of her before she would touch her coffee!" she offered. "Maybe that's what she's missing."

The next day, a staff member brought in a newspaper and put it in Evelyn's spot at the dining table. As Evelyn sat down, he placed a cup of hot coffee in front of her, too. A smile moved across Evelyn's face as she picked up the newspaper in her left hand and began to read. Her right hand reached out and picked up the cup, bringing it to her lips.

Evelyn still liked drinking coffee every morning, but she wanted it a certain way. Even though Evelyn could not communicate her preferences, once the staff met her needs she was able to appreciate the drink. Often, family members or staff assume that people with dementia no longer want or like the things they used to enjoy. For example, if for decades your father had a habit of waking up, reading the newspaper, and then getting dressed for work, he may have difficulty getting ready for the day without the paper. It does not matter if your dad actually reads the paper—what matters is that it is an important part of his routine. The newspaper cues him that it is time to get up and get dressed. The newspaper reminds him that it is time for breakfast. He is better able to go through the steps of the day when something prompts him to get started. When caregivers assume that people with dementia no longer have those individual preferences, some crucial daily cues get lost. When daily cues are lost, so are important self-care actions.

ARTICULATING PREFERENCES

People with dementia often have trouble articulating their preferences, likes, and dislikes. Even though your dad loves reading the paper, he may have trouble telling you that. In fact, because of his cognitive loss, he may not realize that it's missing from his routine. When your dad begins having trouble getting up and preparing for the day ahead, you may assume it is because his dementia has gotten worse. The real reason, however, is that your dad is missing his newspaper—the one thing that cued him to start the day.

A good care community should ask a resident's family members plenty of questions about their loved one. When choosing a dementia care community, learn whether the staff gets to know residents on paper as well as in person. It should be a red flag if a community does not ask the family several questions about a new resident. Questions should be about a person's life growing up, his career, his relationships, his likes and dislikes, his favorite foods, and even potential sources of pain and trauma in his life.

Caregivers should know the answers to the following questions before moving a person with dementia into a community:

- What time does your family member or friend like to wake up?
- What is a normal day like for your family member or friend?
- What did your family member or friend do for a living?
- What level of education did your family member or friend reach?
- What was your family member or friend's life like growing up?

- Who were your family member or friend's biggest influences?
- Who was your family member or friend's spouse or partner? How long have they been together, and is the partner still living?
- Does your family member or friend have children? How many and what are their names?
- Are there any traumas or areas of stress that should never be mentioned?
- What foods does your family member or friend like and dislike?
- What is your family member or friend's bedtime routine like? At what time of day does your family member or friend shower or bathe?
- What types of music does your family member or friend like?
- Does your family member or friend like animals? What types of pets has your family member or friend had?
- What does your family member or friend do for fun?
- Is religion important to your family member or friend?

The questions a community asks may combine both personal care questions (such as questions about bathing and bedtimes) and life history questions. Family caregivers may have difficulty answering some of these questions, especially if the primary caregivers did not live with their parent, partner, or sibling. Before moving a person to a long-term-care community, it may be wise for caregivers to pay close attention to their loved one's routines. When does your mother go to bed? What exactly does she like to do before she falls asleep? Taking note of these things before she needs a care community will make the move easier.

Staff members need to know what to talk to a person about and what to avoid. They need to know their residents well, which comes from understanding both their histories and their care needs. History provides staff members with knowledge about a person's emotional requirements. For example, knowing that a resident was a teacher for 40 years tells the staff a lot about that person. It probably means that she loves kids, will try to look after other residents, and likely enjoys being in charge of groups. This kind of information will help the staff plan her day and find activities to engage and interest her.

Because of the large group of retired teachers in our care community, we planned a trip to a local preschool to read to the children, even though these residents all had moderate to moderately advanced dementia. The minute we got to the school, however, it was almost as though my residents' impairments floated away. They picked up the books the children offered and read them all, showing the pages as they went.

One woman in particular, Dorothy, blew me away with her ability to communicate with the children. "Can I read to the kids?" she asked.

"Sure," I said, hesitating, afraid that she was no longer able to read. I didn't want to hand her the book if she was going to struggle with it. Immediately, however, I felt silly for ever being nervous because Dorothy switched on like a lightbulb.

"Hey kids! This book is about dogs! How many of you have a dog at home?" she asked enthusiastically. Nearly all the kids raised their hands and began to get loud, trying to call out over each other. Dorothy held her hand up in the air to quiet them down. "Wow! That is so great! Let's remember, though, to be quiet when an adult is speaking!" she said, smiling.

Her prowess was that of an expert teacher. Dorothy read aloud to the children, pausing on every page to explain the story. The kids acted engaged and excited. They responded to Dorothy's cues like she had been their teacher all year. Chills ran through my body as I watched her talk to the kids that day. I had never witnessed anything so magical as seeing this woman transform into her old self.

TAKE-AWAY POINTS

We all have our own personal preferences. You can probably think of a few things that you do or enjoy that others do not. Now think about them in terms of dementia caregiving. If no one knew that you slept holding a pillow, how would you communicate this if you had dementia? You are having trouble sleeping, but you aren't quite sure what is different. Maybe the care-community staff members assume you have insomnia. They want to place you on a new medication, but the real solution is simple: you just sleep best with a pillow in your arms.

It may be potentially useful to make note of your own personal preferences. Write them down somewhere, type them up, and save the information in a place that others can find. If something were to happen to you, your loved ones would know best how to care for you. All of your preferences would already be written down, and they would be completed by the best person possible—you.

Personal preferences do not disappear when a person gets dementia. In fact, one could argue that preferences become even more important. Knowing someone's daily routine and habits is vital in securing that person the best possible dementia care. The more that the staff at a dementia care community, day-care facility, or home-care agency know about a person with dementia, the better they are able to care for that individual.

The Cost of Good Hygiene

Good hygiene is an important part of life, especially for people with dementia. Although an adult with dementia could once dress herself, toilet independently, and eat without assistance, as her disease progresses, she is left with nearly no ability to care for her own activities of daily living. She now requires the help of others when it comes to cleanliness and hygiene. When choosing a dementia care community, that hygiene often comes with a large price tag.

Different care communities have different fee structures, but many charge separately for room charges and care charges. When choosing a care community for your parent, partner, child, or friend, research in advance what charges will appear on each bill. Most likely, you'll see a base charge for rent in addition to charges for a resident's care and care products. In many communities, as a person's care needs increase, these care charges grow and are added to a family's bill each month.

"We were never told about this charge," the woman said angrily. "Our aunt wasn't supposed to be charged this much for care! Why are we paying for someone to take her to the bathroom? She used to be able to do that herself!"

Sophia's family was angry, and they had a right to be. They had a hard time understanding why they were paying more now, especially when Sophia had, according to them, been toileting herself independently for years. Now, as Sophia's disease progressed, her care charges increased. On top of her rent for the room, the community now charged Sophia's family for an aide's time to help her use the bathroom each day.

"We were only told about the rent base rate," they argued. "We thought it stopped there!"

Before making any big purchase, you would want to learn more about what is included in the final price. Doing your research and getting a quote on the cost of care will save you a lot of heartache once it comes time to move your family member or friend into a care community. Because pricing varies widely from state to state and country to country, there is no one-size-fits-all cost to living in a dementia care community. For example, the fees for a community in New York City are going to be a lot higher than those for a community in rural North Carolina.

URINATION AND DEFECATION

Urinating and defecating in the wrong place are common behaviors in people with dementia and can be a huge problem for caregivers. Many families cite incontinence as a reason they are looking into long-term care for a loved one—it can be embarrassing to talk about and frustrating to handle.

In dementia care communities, professional caregivers must deal with this constantly. Aides are often assigned specific residents by hallway or by room. These aides "round" and usually check their residents hourly to prevent residents from soiling themselves, going in the wrong spot, or sitting in wet undergarments for long periods of time.

There should never be an inordinate number of residents assigned to any one caregiver—although the exact ratio required in each community varies by state and country. It's important to ask about the community's ratio of aides to residents before choosing it as someone's new home. Residents with dementia require much more care and observation than residents who do not have cognitive impairments, so dementia care communities should have a greater aide-to-resident ratio.

Care communities where residents are not checked frequently or are left in wet undergarments too long can emit a bad odor. In some situations, communities will have to rip up soiled floors to ensure their hallways smell fresh and clean. There is no reason that a dementia care community should smell bad all the time. When searching for the right community, caregivers should look for a place that smells and looks clean—at least a majority of the time. They do need to understand, however, that there are "those days" when a resident has had an accident, and a particular hallway or room smells unpleasant. It is advisable to visit the community twice before choosing it for your parent, partner, child, or friend. With different days come different situations, different smells, and different amounts of activity and cleanliness.

Some residents, no matter what arrangements are made for them, will struggle with the ability to use the bathroom at the right time. Take Shirley, who was notorious in one community for defecating in trash cans. Although it seems odd and unsanitary, Shirley had a lot of trouble finding her room. Instead of looking for the closest bathroom, Shirley found the next best thing—and something that resembled a toilet: a trash can. Shirley ruined a number of trash cans before the staff devised a toileting schedule that worked for her.

Like Shirley, some residents have trouble finding the bathroom or recognizing when it is "time to go." If someone with dementia lives long enough with the disease, that person will have some trouble with incontinence. Many residents in care communities wear disposable adult briefs made specifically for people with incontinence issues. Some care communities provide briefs without charge, others provide briefs and charge for them, and still others require a resident's family to supply briefs. It's a good idea to ask about incontinence products before choosing a specific care community.

BRUSHING TEETH

Giving a person with dementia the opportunity to continue caring for herself is very important. The ability to wake up in the morning, dress herself, brush her own teeth, and get ready are basic activities of daily living. As a person's dementia progresses, however, the ability to accomplish these basic tasks begins to fail. Even though it can be time consuming—and, at times, frustrating—to watch a person with dementia struggle to do the things she used to do, it's imperative that caregivers at least let her try.

As Jennifer got ready for bed, she seemed to be having trouble moving from one step to another. She would turn on the water and then forget to put soap on her hands. She would put soap on her hands, wash them, and then forget to dry them. Jennifer required constant cueing, even though she could do the tasks on her own once she got started.

"Here's the towel," I offered, handing her the washcloth.

"Oh, thank you, dear," she said. Jennifer dried her hands. The process was slow, and I had to be very patient. I did not want to take away Jennifer's abilities and do things for her, although that would have made the bedtime routine much faster.

"Here is your toothbrush," I said, putting toothpaste on it and handing it to her.

"Thank you," she said, accepting the brush. Jennifer paused and looked at the toothbrush for a moment. She took it in her right hand and began brushing her left arm with it.

"Oh, you use the toothbrush like this," I said, surprised, motioning at my own teeth and brushing them with an invisible toothbrush.

"Oh, right," she said. "I guess I'm just tired tonight." Jennifer sighed, trying to make sense of the reason why she had forgotten how to use her toothbrush.

Jennifer required a lot of cueing to get started on a task, but she could do it herself given a push in the right direction. Great caregivers will give their family members or residents time to care for themselves. If I had brushed Jennifer's teeth for her, I would have taken away an instrumental part of her ability to look after her own needs.

Eventually, Jennifer would lose the ability to brush her teeth at all. Because she lived in a care community, an aide would brush her teeth for her. Even though she could not do it herself, her oral care would still need to be seen to.

SHOWERS

Dementia care communities vary in their bathroom setups. For example, while some communities have communal showers, others place showers in the residents' rooms. There is no one "right" layout for a dementia community's bathrooms so long as residents are safe while using them. Care aides help residents take showers or baths, depending on the resident's preference. It is important to let the community's directors know what time of day your family member or friend prefers to bathe.

Find out if you need to supply towels, shampoo, and soaps before moving your parent, partner, child, or friend into a care community. Some places will provide towels but not soap or shampoo. Will the care community do your loved one's laundry? Are they going to supply something if he runs out of it at the last minute? These are important questions to ask when choosing a care community.

SOAP AND DANGEROUS PRODUCTS

Finally, it is imperative that families know what types of products are allowed at their chosen dementia care community. Different states and countries have different regulations about the types of products they allow residents to have. Although it seems bizarre that communities would take products away from residents, it's only for safety's sake. For example, a resident could mistake a toxic shampoo left on a countertop for a beverage. If that resident drinks the shampoo, he could get very sick—or even die. No care community wants that to happen, so many places have specific regulations about what products they allow.

Most communities allow any shampoos or soaps as long as they are under lock and key. Residents in more mild stages of dementia can find this type of security frustrating.

"Why can't you open my closet door? Just leave it open, please!" Ciara cried out. Ciara was upset that we were not allowed to leave her closet open. She was in a mild to moderate stage of dementia, so the fact that she could not open her closet whenever she wanted annoyed her. "I want to get out the clothes I need!" she shouted.

The problem with leaving Ciara's closet open was that her soap and shampoos were inside. Although Ciara did not have a problem using them appropriately, we feared that other residents would get into her closet and get hold of the products. Although it irritated Ciara, protecting the other residents' safety came first.

In some situations, care communities will provide soap or shampoo via automatic dispensers in the bathrooms. Because in many places residents are not allowed to have products on their sinks that could be dangerous if ingested, there has to be another way to store potentially harmful chemicals.

"I just don't understand why my mom can't have soap in her room," Carol argued. "She likes this specific soap, and I want her to have it."

"I know it's frustrating," I tried to explain. "But that's why we have those automatic soap dispensers—it limits the amount of soap that comes out at one time, and we don't have to worry about residents drinking it."

"My mom won't drink soap!" Carol yelled at me. "She's not some kind of idiot!" Carol was beyond angry, and I understood why. What she could not realize, however, was that it was for the other residents' protection. Some residents tended to wander in and out of other people's rooms. Because we could not watch everyone every second of the day, we could not know if a resident with more advanced dementia got her hands on Carol's mother's soap.

Many family members have difficulty understanding why their parent, partner, sibling, or child with dementia cannot have immediate access to the same products that people without dementia can. It seems unfair and cruel, but it's entirely for the residents' protection.

It takes a lot of patience and understanding from family caregivers and care aides alike to provide residents with the best possible hygiene care. Although a person with dementia won't lose the ability to care for himself overnight, as long as he lives with the disease he will need more hands-on care over time. If he resides in a dementia care community, families should be prepared for the cost for his care to increase as his needs increase. Families should also realize that communities differ in the types of products that residents are allowed to have. Recognizing these things, especially when touring potential communities, can save a lot of headache.

16

Move-In Day: Dropping Your Loved One Off

Deciding on a dementia care community for a parent, partner, adult child, sibling, or friend can be stressful and challenging in and of itself. The day a family must leave their loved one at a care community, however, is perhaps even more upsetting. Many caregivers experience immense amounts of guilt over it. They feel as if they are betraying their family member or friend by not caring for him at home and feel terrible forcing that person to relocate.

This is the reality for many family caregivers. There are, however, ways to handle dropping someone off at a care community with grace.

Madeline was not pleased. In fact, she was downright furious. "Open the door!" she screamed, smashing her fists on the glass. "Open this door right now!"

Madeline had just been dropped off at a dementia care community, but her family did not leave with ease. They had turned moving day into a complete disaster by telling Madeline that she had dementia and that she would be permanently living in the community. "Mom, you're here because you are sick, remember?" Madeline's daughter told her. "You have to stay here so that you'll be safe!"

This was not the right thing to tell Madeline. She was now angry, confused, and wanted to leave immediately. Madeline did not believe she was sick—she felt fine! She did not want to be in a locked community where old and ill people lived. She was determined to get outside and get back to her house.

After giving her this information, Madeline's family attempted to leave the community without her. They bolted for the door and ran out before Madeline could catch up with them. The older woman watched as they drove away and continued to beat on the door with closed fists. It took hours to calm Madeline down and get her away from the door.

It was a tragic scene that could have gone differently had Madeline's family known how to handle the conversation. It is important to note, however, that Madeline's reaction is a worst-case scenario: most people with dementia don't act like this upon moving into a new community. Madeline did eventually accept it, but it took longer than her family had expected. Although there is always a risk that a person with dementia will be upset about moving into a community, especially at first, several tactics can help you get through this difficult day without turning it into a traumatic experience for everyone involved.

VISITING AHEAD OF TIME

Madeline's family could have taken her to visit the community ahead of time to get her enthused about her new home. They could have shown her to her new room and presented it with a positive attitude. "Wow, Mom, this is a really nice room," they could have offered. "You have a beautiful view and plenty of space." They could have taken Madeline on a tour of the community, pointing out great spots to relax and enjoy. Perhaps they could have visited the dining area and even tasted some of the food. By making the new environment an exciting and happy one, the family could have easily decreased Madeline's anxiety and anger. Even if Madeline was just seeing the community for the first time on move-in day, if the family had approached the move with positivity, Madeline no doubt would have felt better about it, too.

They could also have let Madeline believe it was *her* idea to move to the community. If they felt she would understand the situation, they could have taken her to a few communities to tour. Maybe Madeline could have helped them decide which community to choose. Like most of us, people with dementia feel good when they are empowered and think they have some control over their own lives.

Madeline could have helped her family move her into the community. She might have carried a couple of pillows inside while her family lugged the bigger items. Or, perhaps she could have stood in the room and directed where furniture should go. She would probably have felt as though she was choosing the move, or at least choosing the way the room would look. People want to feel necessary, and no one wants to feel as though decisions are being made for her.

EMOTIONS SURROUNDING THE MOVE

Madeline's family had a chance to help her look forward to living in the community instead of turning it into a place where "sick people live." They could have presented it as a happy community where she would make many friends. They could have suggested that they chose it because she would enjoy herself there. Many people with dementia in moderate to advanced stages lack the insight to realize there is anything wrong with them or others with dementia. By telling Madeline she was sick, her family put her on the defensive. No one wants to believe she is sick or injured. After she heard that sick people lived there, Madeline became fearful and aggressive. She didn't feel as though she belonged in that environment, so she immediately began to fight back and tried to leave.

Telling Madeline that she would have to "stay there to be safe" and that she "lived there now" was also a mistake. By telling her these things, they put a timeline on Madeline's stay—they made the stay permanent. Putting this timeline on her stay overwhelmed and confused Madeline. Many people with dementia lose their ability to understand the passage of time. Two days can feel like an eternity, but two years can fly by. When asking those with dementia how long they have lived in a community, do not expect an accurate answer. Many people will say things like "I have been here for three days" when they have actually lived there for six months. When Madeline learned the move was permanent, she panicked. That would be scary for anyone, but it is particularly terrifying for someone who does not understand the concept of time.

Another way to handle moving day would have been to provide Madeline with something to do once she arrived. Maybe she could have taken part in a meaningful activity, or perhaps her family could have introduced her to a new friend. While Madeline was happily engaged, they could have said goodbye for the day and left quietly.

The worst-case scenario is that a family member or friend with dementia absolutely does not want to move—and understands that he is about to do so. If a person with dementia knows that he is leaving a home behind, he may become combative. While taking the above steps are important, sometimes a person just refuses to relocate, and he will not make the process any easier for his family. The best thing to do in this situation is to distract him: Get the person with dementia inside the community, get him involved in a task or activity, and get the staff involved. Enjoy a meal with him at the community or help him begin a painting exercise. Once that person is engaged and active, it is time for the family to leave.

Although it seems cruel, it is much better than telling a person with dementia that he "lives there now" or suggesting that he is there because of an illness. Sometimes, families try other suggestions, like telling the person with dementia that he is at the community for a doctor's appointment or an extended physical therapy stay. Often, these techniques do work, because the person with dementia does not feel as though he is stuck at the new community. Eventually, as day or weeks pass, he will adjust, and the agitation over the move will subside.

People with dementia take varying amounts of time to adjust to life at a new community. Some people adapt immediately, while others can take days or even weeks. I once had a family member tell me, "Well, you've had my mom for three days, so I don't understand why she seems agitated when I visit." Three days is not enough time for most people to adjust to anything at all. Think about your own moves: Did you immediately become comfortable with your surroundings when you relocated to a new place? Probably not. With that said, most new residents with dementia do not take more than a week to become settled. It's important to note, too, that once a person with dementia is settled into a good community, he should not be relocated.

VISITING RIGHT AFTER THE MOVE

Some dementia community leaders will recommend that family members not visit a resident right after the move. Truly, though, there is no right or wrong answer as to when a person should visit. Some family members visit right away, while others wait a week or two to let their parent, partner, or child adjust. This is an entirely personal decision. Some residents do better when they are given the space to get used to their new home. Others crave the comfort of seeing their families every day.

SECOND-GUESSING THE MOVE

If the first day at a dementia care community fails to go smoothly, families will often second-guess their decision. Some will say things like "My mom isn't like the other people here," or "She isn't ready for this type of care." Typically, families overreact out of fear—they suddenly worry that their loved one is not ready for dementia community care. A catastrophic reaction, such as a person with dementia screaming, crying, or arguing, tends to send many family members into panic mode. They immediately jump to the conclusion that every day will be like this and that they must move their parent or sibling out of community care.

It is so important to give a person with dementia time to adjust to her new environment. The first day of any move will never go perfectly. Let the professionals at the community evaluate the new resident and watch her behavior over the first few days. Although you may be tempted to turn right around and move her out of community care, it's best to wait at least a few weeks before making any rash decisions.

Joyce was doing really well at her community. She had good friends, knew how to find her room, and enjoyed going on outings with the staff. All things considered, Joyce was thriving. Still, her family was looking for a less expensive option for her care. "This place is really expensive, and one of the nearby dementia communities is a lot cheaper," they argued.

Eventually, the family decided to move Joyce. She had lived in the first community for a couple of years and was incredibly angry about being moved. After the new move, Joyce's dementia began to progress much faster than before. Her walking, speaking, and understanding all got a lot worse. She became confused about the layout of the new location. She wasn't sure where her room was anymore, and the people she normally saw each day were absent. Even though she had Alzheimer's disease, Joyce had adjusted to the people and patterns in her first community. The move disoriented her completely: she no longer knew where she was or what she was doing.

In some situations a move from one community to another is unavoidable. Be it because of money; family relocation; or another immediate, major issue, some people will need to move between dementia communities. It is important to remember, however, that people with dementia do take time to adjust to new things. Once they adjust to and enjoy the things and people that a community offers, they can find it difficult to readjust to a new place. In Joyce's case, the change set her back. Again, although a move may have to happen for a specific reason, try to remember the importance of avoiding another relocation, if possible.

REMAINING POSITIVE

Families can handle move-in day in numerous ways. If a family is positive and excited about the move, a person with dementia will most likely feel the same. If a family approaches the move with caution, anxiety, and sadness, a person with dementia will probably also feel distressed. It is imperative that caregivers remain positive, even when the day becomes very stressful. People with dementia do not lose their ability to understand other people's emotions. If anything, they probably become even more responsive to them. In order to handle move-in day with grace, the family must first decide to be happy about the relocation themselves.

17

Saying Goodbye for the Day

One of the hardest things about visiting a parent, partner, child, or friend in a dementia care community is saying goodbye for the day. Many visitors struggle with this. In an effort to tell the truth, family members will often tell their loved ones that they are "going home" after a visit. This typically begins a negative chain of events.

WHAT HOME MEANS

For many people, especially romantic partners, "home" is a loaded word. When people with dementia hear the word "home," they typically think of the house they lived in with family members or a spouse—not their current long-term-care community. Although adult children can sometimes use the phrase "going home" without an issue, many spouses cannot exercise this same privilege.

If your family member or friend is not too advanced into dementia and is able to understand that you need to leave, then it's acceptable to announce that you are going home. Regardless, exercise caution when using this phrase, especially when your family member first moves to a new community. It's important to test the waters and see how she reacts when you exit the community for the day.

"My mom keeps saying that she wants to go home!" Eva complained. "She's been here for a month, and every time I see her, she asks to go home!"

Eva could not understand why, after all this time, her mother, Crystal, still asked about going home. What she didn't realize, however, was that Crystal never talked about home with anyone else.

Seeing Eva, though, reminded Crystal of home. Crystal's daughter was leaving for the day, so why couldn't they leave together?

Eva was so convinced that her mother hated the care community that she considered moving her out. It was not until she sat in another room and watched her mother eat dinner, happily chatting with other residents, that she realized her own presence probably caused Crystal's obsession with returning home.

When Eva wasn't there, Crystal never mentioned wanting to go home. But when her daughter showed up and mentioned "home," Crystal wanted to go, too.

When significant others with dementia hear their partner is leaving, they often head for the door as well. Consider parties or events you attended together in the past. When you announced that it was "time to go home," you probably both left the event together. This phrase still prompts a person with dementia to believe that you are *both* leaving. It's understandable, then, why your loved one with dementia might get upset and angry when you tell her you are leaving, and she is not allowed to go with you.

James held his wife's hand as they strolled down the hallway of the dementia care community. Charlotte had Alzheimer's disease, but James was dutiful and loving nonetheless. He came to see her at least once a day, and he would always stay for hours at a time. It was clear that the couple cared for each other above anything else. Even if Charlotte fell asleep, James would sit beside her, quietly holding her hand.

When it was time for James to leave for the day, though, he had a lot of difficulty. Instead of telling her that he would see her soon or had a few errands to run, he would tell her that he was "going home."

"Home? Okay, let's go," Charlotte would shrug, heading toward the door with him.

"No, Charlotte, you live here now." James would shake his head, trying to explain. "You have to stay here. Your room is right down the hall."

Immediately, Charlotte would become confused, angry, and devastated. "Why are you saying these mean things to me, James? Why won't you let me come home with you?" she would tearfully plead.

It was a terrible scene to watch, but it happened nearly every time James visited. Although the reaction was always awful, he consistently announced to Charlotte that he was "going home." He was not trying to be cruel, but it was as though he did not understand what else he could do. James had never lied to his wife, and he did not intend to start now, even though he caused her a great deal of anguish in the process of trying to be truthful.

Eventually, after they fought for 15 minutes or so, he would leave for the day. Charlotte would spend the next two hours walking the halls of the community, tears in her eyes. Although she would eventually forget her distress, she wouldn't start feeling better until after she went to bed. The situation started all over again the next day.

James was a wonderful and loving partner to his wife, but he did not understand how to exit the community without creating a confusing and upsetting situation. Some of the following techniques might have allowed him to say goodbye without an issue.

STEPS FOR EXITING WITHOUT A FIGHT

First, unless this person is your spouse, try letting your family member or friend know that you are going home. As an adult child, you may find success in announcing that you are going home for the day. If this person is your spouse and he's confused about where he lives, do not attempt this method.

If telling your parent, sibling, or friend you are "going home" does not produce a positive result, tell him you have to run some errands. This should not feel like a lie. At some point in the future, you'll no doubt need to run errands. Exiting by suggesting that you have to go to the grocery store, visit the bank, or see another friend is probably true. You are not saying that you are "going home," and therefore, the possibility of hurt feelings is less. This method should work for most families without any issues.

For some with dementia, of course, that method will not work. Your family member or friend may suggest going with you. He says he enjoys running errands, and it would be nice to get out for a little while. Maybe you suggest that you "do not have enough room in the car" or that you'll be back soon. Perhaps you have a meeting to go to, and it just would not be appropriate for him to come along. Maybe you are picking up a surprise for him (you can actually do that!), and you do not want him to know what it is. As you can see, there are a number of ways to avoid telling someone that you are "going home" for the day. The key is to remain creative and kind when finding a way to extract yourself.

If your mom, for example, asks why she "has to stay here," you can also give a number of positive responses. The doctor, nurse, or other staff members can assist with this. Maybe she has a doctor's appointment today, and this is where it is. You could also suggest that this is where she will be eating breakfast, lunch, or dinner. If the next meal is coming up soon, this is a great time to exit the community. Maybe you can suggest to your mom that you are dropping her off at the community so she can lead an activity for the other residents. This works particularly well if your mom is used to being in charge of groups. Note that none of these statements need to feel like a lie for either party.

Another easy way to say goodbye for the day is to get your family member or friend involved in an activity or event happening at the community. Maybe a volunteer is coming in to sing for the residents, or perhaps a few of the residents are arranging flowers. If your family member is happy and interested in a new activity, you shouldn't have difficulty leaving. You will probably feel better, too, knowing that she is having a good time.

If all else fails, ask for help. Do not let your need to leave for the day cause a fight, and certainly do not avoid visiting because you dread the moment you have to leave again. The staff at the community are there to help both you and the residents. Pick a staff member you trust and let him or her know ahead of time that you will be leaving. The staff can help to keep your family member engaged or even provide a hand to hold as you exit. No matter what, assure your parent, partner, child, or friend that you'll be back to visit soon—and then follow through on that promise.

Exiting for the day after visiting a loved one with dementia in a care community can be a challenge. It's important to remember that people with dementia live there for a reason: It is a safe, comfortable environment, full of positive stimulation. The staff is available 24 hours a day, seven days a week. Although providing care for a person with dementia at home is noble, it is not the only way to be a wonderful caregiver.

PART IV

RELATIONSHIPS AND DEMENTIA

18

The Importance of Friendship for People Who Have Dementia

Many people assume that residents in dementia care communities do not make real friendships because they cannot remember each other. In a way, this is partly true: People with dementia don't always remember each other. They may not remember names, but they often recognize relationships and understand connections, love, and kindness. Even when a person with dementia does not know a friend's name, she still *knows* that friend. The ability to recognize a personal connection with someone lasts long into dementia's damage to the brain.

Long-term-care communities are unique in allowing people with dementia to make and maintain friendships. In fact, this is perhaps one of the best reasons to choose such care for a parent, partner, sibling, or friend. A person with dementia will enjoy a level of interaction in a dementia care community that she wouldn't get at home. When residents with dementia are surrounded with people their age and cognitive level, friendships blossom.

Many people with moderate or even moderately advanced dementia are able to make and maintain new friendships. Although a person with dementia may not be able to recall another person's name, that doesn't mean she is unable to recognize and establish a true connection with her.

The roommates were inseparable. If one was sleeping, the other was sleeping. If one was on her way to the dining room, the other was right beside her. Vera and Beth were the best of friends. Vera was not as advanced into Alzheimer's disease as Beth, but the two knew each other—there was no doubt about that. Vera knew Beth's name, while Beth did not actually seem to know Vera's. Beth often referred to Vera only as "my roommate," but that distinction worked well for the pair.

"Hey! That seat is saved for my roommate!" Beth often called out to a resident who had taken Vera's seat on their couch. Granted, it was not actually "their" couch, but if the pair sat anywhere, they sat on the same two-seater sofa.

"Oh, don't worry, Beth, I'll just sit over here," Vera would offer.

"No, no, this is your seat, and this knucklehead is sitting in it!" Beth would hiss, pointing at the resident who had adopted Vera's seat.

Whenever an outing took place, Vera ensured that Beth was beside her. "Where's Beth?" she would ask. "She likes ice cream outings, too. I had better go get her!" Vera would go back to the couch to get Beth. The pair would ride on the first two seats of the bus, and Vera would always help Beth up the stairs of the vehicle.

Beth needed Vera for reminders and assistance. Vera leaned on Beth mostly for friendship, because Beth was unable to provide many cues or reminders due to her advancing Alzheimer's. The two widowed women had loving family members, but their families had lives of their own and could not visit too often. In lieu of family, they had each other.

One day, Vera's family decided to move her to a new community. They were relocating and wanted to move her, too. "We aren't worried," the family said. "Vera will eventually forget who her friends are at this community, anyway." I feared what would happen to Beth once Vera moved. Beth relied on Vera's cues and directions to get through the day. She needed her best friend beside her.

The day Vera moved, something changed in Beth. She no longer fought for that couch seat. Often, Beth did not even sit on the couch they used to share. Instead, she migrated from seat to seat, almost aimlessly. Although she could not explain what was missing, something was clearly wrong. Something had changed about her day.

"We'll tell her that Vera is on vacation," the staff agreed, planning ahead in case Beth asked about her friend. It would have been heartbreaking to tell Beth the real truth.

Beth became focused on physical things, like the missing furniture in her bedroom that she once shared with Vera. "What happened to the furniture in here?" she asked. And then, concerned, she turned to me. "Is someone going to sleep in here with me tonight?" Tears welled up in my eyes as I realized that she did not want to be alone.

Beth never asked about Vera, probably because she could not quite place the loss. We found her a new roommate, someone who could also provide cues and direction, but it was not the same. Although the new roommate was kind, the pair did not connect on the same level that Beth and Vera had.

While Beth could not quite place Vera when she was no longer physically present, it did not mean that Beth would not recognize Vera immediately whenever she saw her. Even in a large crowd of residents, Beth could find and point out her friend. Beth didn't know Vera's name, but she knew that Vera was her friend and her roommate. The ability to recognize a person is preserved long into the progression of Alzheimer's disease.

Melissa, like all the residents in her dementia care community, did not know my name. Even though I wore a name badge at the community, Melissa never bothered to read it. None of the residents knew my name, although all of them recognized me as a staff member. Interestingly, however, Melissa assigned me a name, "Susan." Even in a large crowd of residents and staff members, Melissa would seek me out. Often, she would pass other staff members, looking only for me. "Susan, I need your help with something," she would say.

For Melissa, our relationship changed from day to day or even hour to hour. Depending on the day, Melissa would believe that I was her college friend, her student, her work colleague, or even a professor at her college. The relationship always changed, but my name always stayed the same. After some time, I actually began answering to "Susan" because I knew that Melissa was calling out for me.

Of course, I never corrected Melissa. There was no point in telling her that my name was Rachael because, really, it didn't matter. What mattered most was that Melissa knew me in some fashion. She knew that I was friendly and helpful, and so she created a relationship with me based on whatever her brain told her that day. It always fascinated me to see what relationship we would have, and I waited for her cues. If she thought I was her work colleague, I would "assign" her some tasks to do. If she believed we were students in college, I would ask her to join me at the next activity, telling her that it was time for class.

The relationship—the friendship—is what made Melissa's day more meaningful. Even though she created our relationship anew each day, she recognized me as a person she could trust. In each case, whether I was a student, a colleague, a teacher, or a friend, I was someone she looked for. I was honored to receive such a name, even if it was not my real one.

One of the most wonderful things about a long-term-care community is that residents are able to connect with one another. As in any community, some people are not going to mesh well. But when residents do get along, the outcome can be magical. Just as in the story about Beth and Vera, many residents rely on others not just for friendship but for help and guidance.

Patrick stopped by my office and looked at me. "Can you do me a favor?" he asked.

"Of course," I said. "What is it?"

Patrick handed me his cane and explained, "I want to give this to my good friend, Paul." Patrick and Paul sat at the same table in the dining room and had struck up quite a friendship. Although Paul was more advanced in dementia than Patrick, the pair had bonded over talking about work and family.

"He's my best friend here and I want to show him that," Patrick said. "Can you write on the cane, 'For my friend, Paul, from your friend, Patrick'?"

Paul and Patrick were in different stages of dementia, but they still connected with one another. Often, however, people of similar cognitive groups will find each other. For example, all of the residents who spend most of their days walking up and down the hallway will tend to group together. Because they are all out and about—and likely at a similar stage of dementia—they get along well. People of higher functioning levels will also pair off because they are able to converse with one another. Some of the best interactions, though, come about when a person functioning at a higher level helps another person who is deeper into dementia. Some residents will cut up food for others in the dining room, try to help another person stand or walk, or even assist another resident with an article of clothing, such as helping someone put on a jacket. People of higher functioning levels are often able to recognize that others need assistance and are more than happy to provide it. And for the people of lower cognitive functioning, the help that other residents provide is invaluable.

As the story goes, Vera never forgot her friend Beth. "Oh, I hope I get back there to see Beth soon," she would say. Apparently, she never forgot about her past community, even late into her disease. Because Vera had met Beth at a crucial time in her life, perhaps before her Alzheimer's disease had progressed too far, she was able to retain memories of Beth's friendship. In fact, she was even able to recall Beth's name. It was said that Vera believed that one day, she would be moving back to the old community. "I cannot wait to get back there and see my room and my friends," she would say. "Everyone was so nice."

Because people with dementia are at a high risk for depression, for them, making connections with others who have dementia is invaluable. Humans still desire friendship and love, even in the midst of cognitive loss.

19

Sex and Partnership in a Dementia Community

Although many people feel uncomfortable talking about emotional and physical relationships between older adults, the reality is that love and sex do not stop at a certain age. These things do not cease because a person gets dementia, either. They become more challenging when dementia enters the picture, but they still influence many people's lives.

Having dementia does not mean that a person loses the desire or ability to maintain a romantic relationship. For many people with dementia, romantic companionship is still incredibly important. Numerous types of romantic relationships can begin between residents at senior-living communities. While some are physical in nature, others are not. Caregivers can significantly improve their parents', siblings', or friends' lives by accepting their romantic relationships with others.

NEW ROMANCE BETWEEN RESIDENTS

In some cases, people in dementia care communities will partner up. These partnerships may be fleeting, as some residents will constantly forget who their partner is. Other partnerships will remain in place for long periods of time. In these situations, it's up to families to support their family member's decision to be in a relationship. This is a frustrating and embarrassing topic for many people to discuss, particularly if you're caring for your parent. Recognize that the staff at the community expect these kinds of relationships to begin and do not judge you or your parent for allowing them to continue.

Michelle had never seemed to notice Russell before. They had both lived at the community for years, but suddenly, it appeared the two were a couple. Before she noticed Russell, Michelle mostly kept to herself. She was a kind and incredibly well-dressed woman of 81 years, but she never wanted to join in community activities or outings. "Oh, no, honey, I think I'll just stay behind here," Michelle would say when asked about going out for lunch or ice cream.

As soon as she met Russell, everything changed. The pair could be found strolling the hallways together, hand in hand. They did everything together, including going on outings. Russell had never been much for trips outside the community either, but together the pair was up for any and all adventures. It was clear to everyone that they brought out the best in each other.

Michelle's daughters were more than happy about her new relationship. "Mom is doing so well now! We love that she's become close with Russell," they explained. The same could not be said for Russell's daughter, however. She was obviously distraught over her father's relationship with a woman who was not her mother. Even though Russell's wife had passed away years before, Russell's daughter didn't think her father should have any more romantic partners.

Eventually, Russell's daughter decided to move him to a new community. Although she claimed that it was because the new community was closer to her home, it likely had something to do with Russell's relationship. Immediately after Russell moved out, Michelle's attitude changed. "He'll be back, I know it," she would say. It was clear that, even though she had dementia, Michelle spent quite a long time mourning the loss of her boyfriend.

Michelle and Russell made a fantastic pair, but unfortunately, Russell's daughter didn't see it that way. She was bothered, like many family caregivers, by her father carrying on a romantic relationship in a senior-living community. What she could not understand, however, was that her dad still needed love, companionship, and affection. Russell was an adult who, even though he had dementia, was still capable of making his own decisions regarding companionship. Russell had chosen another cognitively impaired adult with whom he could have a consensual relationship. Moving to a new community most likely affected his mental state. He was probably more confused and lonely than before. Dementia and depression often go hand in hand, and encouraging positive relationships between residents can be a great way to combat this.

Although it is your prerogative to try and prevent your loved one's relationships with others, it is best to accept that you cannot truly stop him from engaging with other residents. You are not there all day, every day, and your family member or friend with dementia is going to do what he wants to do. Remind yourself that your family member is an adult and that it is not your job to manage his relationships with other adults—even though he is cognitively impaired.

MARRIAGE AND DEMENTIA

One of the biggest challenges that some caregivers encounter is seeing their married family member or partner begin a relationship with another resident. Under normal circumstances, a married adult having a relationship with a person other than her spouse is usually considered adultery. However, dementia is not a normal circumstance. As always, it is imperative to embrace the reality of the person with dementia. Some people with dementia are unable to remember that they are married, while others believe that another resident is, in fact, their real spouse.

Gloria and Joe were inseparable. The pair did very well together because they shared the same level of cognitive functioning. The only problem, however, was that Joe was still married. Joe's wife, Sue, visited the community often. She knew about Joe's relationship with Gloria, but there wasn't much she could do. Even though Joe enjoyed his real wife's visits, he always went back to Gloria's side after Sue left the community for the day.

In Joe's mind, Gloria was his wife. He saw Gloria every day, her room was next to his, and they sat at the same dining room table. Joe knew who Sue was when she came to visit, too, but his confusion seemed to wax and wane with the passing hours. Joe also seemed to believe that Sue and Gloria were the same person, and in his world, that made sense. Both Gloria and Sue had blond hair and a similar body type. When Sue was not there, Joe's brain made sense of her absence, and his new home, by making Gloria his wife. Although it confused outside parties, in Joe and Gloria's world their relationship made perfect sense.

Joe would introduce Gloria as his wife to staff members. "Where's my wife?" he would ask, and the staff would point to Gloria. If Sue was there, the staff members would point to Sue. Because of Joe's memory impairment, he was unable to make this connection. To him, both women were his wife, and both women brought him happiness.

Sue was surprisingly tolerant and even accepting of her husband's relationship with Gloria. She understood that his brain forced him to live in a different world now than hers. In some ways, Sue was even thankful for Gloria—Gloria kept Joe company when she could not be present. Although Sue found it hard at times, she knew Joe loved her more than anything. In fact, he loved her so much that his brain created a copy of her when she could not be there.

Not everyone can be as accepting of a loved one's relationship as Sue was with Joe. Sue's ability to turn her husband's relationship into a positive event made their lives less dramatic. Instead of being upset and jealous, she understood that her husband had dementia. Sue knew that Joe was confused about his relationship with her because she was not always by his side. Sue decided to be happy and accepting, rather than angry, that this confusion had occurred.

SEX AND DEMENTIA

In dementia care, marriage can sometimes become a confusing topic. When one spouse has dementia, even the line between sexual consent and sexual assault can blur. People with dementia, especially later in the disease process, may not have the ability to consent to sexual activity. As a result, married couples may need to reevaluate their physical relationship because of dementia's impact. A spouse used to having a regular sexual routine can find this challenging.

Ken and Mary-Lou had been married for 50 years. Their relationship had always been happy and loving and so had their sex life. As they aged, both began to have some cognitive loss, but Mary-Lou's dementia was significantly worse than her husband's. Even though they moved to the same room in the same community, Ken did not need the same level of care that his wife did.

Mary-Lou was confused. At times, she was not quite sure who her husband actually was. Ken, however, always knew who Mary-Lou was and wished to have the same relationship with her that he had always had. The problem was that Mary-Lou no longer had the ability to consent to sexual activity. She could not really say yes or no because of the way dementia had impaired her brain.

A few times the staff had to actually separate the couple. Because Mary-Lou was no longer sure how to engage in sexual activity, her husband was pushing her into sex without her consent. Although it was awkward, the staff did their best to keep an eye on the couple's physical encounters.

The issue of sexual consent is an important and confusing part of dementia care. It is not a black-and-white issue. Although Ken and Mary-Lou had had a fulfilling sex life in the past, Mary-Lou's new brain state prevented her from enjoying or understanding what was occurring. At times, she wasn't even sure who her husband was. It became an issue, then, of timing. At times, Mary-Lou could consent to and enjoy sexual activity with her husband. At other times, Mary-Lou was not capable of consent at all. Like Mary-Lou, some people with dementia do not necessarily have the ability to understand what is going on before, during, or after sex.

HOMOSEXUALITY

Interestingly, some people in dementia care communities who once identified as heterosexual may end up identifying otherwise. This is not because being around the same sex "turns" a person gay. It may happen because a person has been a closeted homosexual his whole life. Now, with dementia, his filter is gone, and he seems to be attracted to the same sex. It's doubtful that anyone with dementia would come out and say, "I'm gay now," but a person may begin acting as though he is. A significant number of people in senior care were probably told, when young, that they were not supposed to be homosexual. Now, in dementia care, they are finding their true selves.

Ellen had always been a lesbian but had never told anyone. She had grown up in the 1940s, a time when people did not often come out as homosexual. She did what society expected of her: she married a man, had children, and lived out her life. Now that Ellen had Alzheimer's disease, though, the part of her brain that told her to hide her homosexuality was gone.

The staff was slightly confused when Ellen began holding hands with another female resident in the community. They were even more surprised when they spotted the pair kissing in the hallway. "I thought Ellen was married to a guy!" one staff member commented.

RESPECT

Although a relationship between older adults is an issue that many families do not enjoy discussing, it is important to have this discussion. Because the people in senior communities are adults, they are able to decide with whom they will or will not have a physical relationship. In most communities, staff will notify families immediately following a sexual encounter between their family member and another person.

Family caregivers then bear the difficult task of deciding to encourage or dissuade this relationship between their family member and another person. One of the best ways to decide this is to talk to the staff at the dementia care community. If a relationship is positive, full of joy and consent, caregivers may find that respecting their loved one's desire to engage in that relationship is the best thing to do. Even if that relationship is uncomfortable to think about or discuss, emotional and physical relationships between residents can be influential, powerful, and loving.

20

Trouble with Other Residents

People living in dementia care communities benefit from having others with dementia surrounding them. This gives many residents a chance to make friends, create relationships, and have meaningful interactions each day. Of course, it also leads to plenty of opportunities for residents to bicker and disagree with each other.

Like everyone, those with dementia have certain people they prefer over others. Unlike everyone else, however, people with dementia face an added struggle: cognitive loss. This may cause residents to snap at each other, argue, and even start physical confrontations.

"Give me back my blanket! That is my blanket, and you stole it from me!" Arlene cried out, trying to snatch her handwoven blanket back from Marla's grasp.

"This ain't your blanket!" Marla yelled. "My momma made this blanket for me, and if you try and take it I'll slap you right across the face!"

Marla was not just threatening Arlene with words. Marla was the type of woman who meant what she said, and the staff knew she would slap Arlene without hesitation. I quickly intervened and assessed the situation. I knew the blanket did belong to Arlene, but Marla had a tendency to enter other residents' rooms and take their belongings. Marla believed that the entire community belonged to her and her family, and there was no use in trying to convince her otherwise.

Marla went into other people's rooms so often that many of the residents actually began to remember her. "Hey! That's the lady who takes my stuff! Get her out of here!" some of the residents would yell when they saw her approach.

In order to get the blanket back without confrontation, I calmly asked Marla to join me outside. It was over 90 degrees Fahrenheit in the courtyard, and I knew Marla wouldn't care about that blanket for too long in that kind of heat. We talked for a couple of minutes outside. "Hey, Marla, do you want that blanket?" I asked. "It's pretty warm out here!"

"No, it's too hot for this thing." Marla shook her head, handing me the blanket.

I eventually returned the blanket to Arlene. That blanket, however, was just a small victory in the ongoing battle of dealing with Marla's behavior. It was a shame, but because she posed a physical threat to residents Marla was eventually moved out of the community.

Marla's case is an extreme example. Our staff could not keep her or the other residents safe, especially when she angered them so often. All of the residents' family members knew her, too, and many of them probably feared what she'd do next. Marla was an incredibly confrontational person, so it was tough to have her around so many other people.

When a resident constantly gets into trouble with others, alternative placement may be in order. Typically, it takes multiple complaints or a serious incident before a resident must leave the community. Because it's so hard for some families to find dementia community placement, many communities hesitate to force anyone to leave. If the reasons are serious enough, though, a community can relocate a resident even if the family is against it.

In many cases, disputes between residents arise because one or both of them has a medical issue that hasn't been solved. For example, many residents' behaviors change when they have urinary tract infections, or UTIs. UTIs affect people with dementia very differently than they do people with normal cognitive functioning. UTIs commonly cause increased confusion, agitation, anxiety, anger, and sudden mood swings in people with dementia. Most UTIs clear up quickly with medication, and typically any issues between residents dissipate.

WHAT YOU CAN DO

If an issue between residents occurs while you are visiting, try not to get involved. Something you say or do could anger another resident further, and you may find yourself a target. For example, if you are visiting your father in his dementia care community and you see that another resident, Mrs. Blackwell, is not her usual pleasant self, let a manager know. If she and your father have always gotten along well but she now seems aggressive and upset, this could signal something seriously wrong with Mrs. Blackwell's health. Sometimes families notice behavioral changes before staff members, especially if their loved one has close friends in the community. And, if another resident acts aggressively toward you or your family member with dementia, seek help immediately. Do not attempt to calm the person down or prevent a verbal fight if you don't know the best way to proceed.

Hattie stood at the door, smashing it with her fists. "Open this damn door right now!" she screamed. Every once in a while, Hattie would throw herself into a rage regarding the door. Generally, she was very pleasant, but it did not take much to agitate her. One of Hattie's biggest pet peeves had to do with her personal space. She needed her personal space. Any time another resident or staff member attempted to calm her down by getting too close, Hattie just became angrier.

Jason, a family member of a different resident, decided to take matters into his own hands. He had never met Hattie and didn't know anything about her—including her need for personal space.

"Hey, Hattie! What's going on?" he asked jubilantly, trying to put a smile on her face. He reached out to touch her shoulder in an attempt to send a message of comfort.

She turned on her heels and faced him. "What's going on? What's going on! Can't you see I'm trying to go home and no one will let me! You are all going to hell!" Hattie screamed in his face, raising her hand in the air like she was going to slap him. A staff member quickly ran to Jason's aid and prevented a physical assault from occurring.

Although Jason tried to help, he just made the situation a lot worse. Jason didn't know Hattie, so he didn't understand the best way to approach her. People with dementia require special attention and care. Jason's approach might have worked with someone who was more cognitively aware, but his touch and his calm voice were not what Hattie wanted. Instead of intervening the way he did, Jason should have gone to find a staff member. Staff members are better able to handle these kinds of situations. It is a much greater liability for a family member to try and calm a resident or break up a potential fight.

RECURRING PROBLEMS WITH RESIDENTS

If an issue between your parent, partner, child, or friend with dementia and another resident seems ongoing, talk to the executive director, or whoever runs the community. It is not fair for your family member to live in a community—and for you to pay for it—where another person continually bothers him. Ongoing issues are rare, although they do sometimes occur between roommates who just don't get along. Usually, one of the roommates desires more space than the other. For example, if Milton feels very protective over his room, he may not understand why his roommate, Matthew, is always there. Milton believes the room belongs only to him, so he picks verbal fights when Matthew enters the room. Ongoing squabbles like these do not happen often, mostly because of the nature of dementia. Many residents lack the ability to remember small quarrels that they have with others, but they may recall that another resident upsets them on a regular basis.

Marie was terrified of Louis. They had argued one time, and he had threatened to hit her. Although Marie's short-term memory was very poor, she could still recall a strong emotion like fear. Marie still harbored a lot of bad feelings for Louis—even if Louis did not feel the same. In fact, Louis seemed to have forgotten the confrontation completely. Still, Marie refused to enter a room where he was sitting unless she had a staff member by her side. This became an issue because Louis liked to sit in common areas.

Instead of getting involved in the dispute, Marie's daughter did the right thing: she talked to the staff. They were able to assure her that Louis had not made any threats for quite some time but that they would continue to look out for Marie's health and safety. Marie's daughter also always greeted Louis with kindness and let her mother see this. Louis always responded positively, and Marie's fear of the man began to dissipate. As the months went by, her fear subsided. Eventually, she was able to enter rooms where Louis sat without an issue.

Marie's daughter dealt with the problem by employing two important techniques: talking to upper-level staff members and showing kindness and courtesy to Louis. Marie saw these positive interactions, and they helped her get over the issue.

Although many people with dementia get along wonderfully, the chance always exists that two people will not connect. If an issue develops between your family member or friend with dementia and another person, remember to take the high road. Instead of intervening and potentially making the problem worse, look to the staff to help ease your concerns. Recognize that two people with dementia—even if they are the same age and gender and share similar backgrounds—are not going to have the same experience with cognitive loss. Remembering this can make your interactions with other people who have dementia a lot easier.

21

Agitation in the Evening: Preventing and Coping with Sundowning

Sundowning describes a pattern of behavior that some people with dementia exhibit in the late afternoon and evening. Although dementia-related agitation can happen at any time during the day, most seems to occur as the sun begins to set. Many caregivers have seen firsthand how quickly a person with dementia's emotions can change, especially from morning to night. An increase in agitation, irritability, depression, or aggression can occur in even the kindest, most well-tempered of people.

CAUSES OF SUNDOWNING

Among a few competing ideas about why sundowning happens, the most accurate reason is likely to be this: sundowning happens because people with dementia, like most adults, tire out as the day progresses. Throughout the day they experience stressors; deal with changes in routine, medication, and food; and interact with other people. Whereas people without dementia can announce that they are exhausted and need to be left alone, people with dementia may have trouble expressing the same sentiment. People with dementia also become overwhelmed more quickly than people without dementia. Crowded areas or loud and continuous noises can irritate adults with cognitive loss. This is why, particularly in dementia care communities, sundowning is a common syndrome. There are plenty of people to interact with, a high level of entertainment and noise, and a number of visitors in and out the doors each day.

Meredith was beyond upset. Screaming hysterically as we wheeled her down the hallway, she reached out to grab onto anything she could. "Get away from me!" she yelled at everyone she saw.

This version of Meredith was very different from how she had behaved earlier. Children from a local school had come in to visit with the residents for Halloween. The residents loved listening to the kids sing songs. "Come here," Meredith had said, tears of joy in her eyes as she had reached her arms out to the small children. Nearly 30 kids had hugged her, one at a time, as they left the building for the afternoon.

Meredith had enjoyed every second of the children's performance. It was not until over an hour after they had left that her exhaustion and panic had set in. The afternoon performance had collided with her sundowning. Now, she was overwhelmed, tired, and beyond aggravated.

In order to calm her, the staff members wheeled her down the hallway to a quiet space. For safety, someone had to stay in the room with Meredith so she didn't try to stand up and fall out of her wheelchair. This staff member sat behind Meredith's chair so that she could not see that someone else was in the room. It took a few minutes in a quiet space, but Meredith eventually calmed down.

It was wonderful that Meredith was able to interact with the children, but the visiting session had probably gone on too long. More than double the number of people had been in the community than usual, causing double the amount of commotion. Because it was late afternoon and Meredith had had an exciting day, she was exhausted. Someone without dementia would have been able to say, "I'm feeling tired and I think that I just need to spend some time by myself." As a person with dementia, however, Meredith broke down. In order to avoid this extreme sundowning episode, staff members probably should have moved Meredith to a quiet space immediately after the kids left so she could recuperate.

Families can experience a great deal of stress when visiting a parent, partner, child, or friend in a dementia care community. A family member with dementia who is sundowning can make it significantly more challenging. In order to avoid a sundowning episode, it's best if caregivers visit before 4:00 p.m. or so. Many people with dementia fare just fine in the late afternoons, but some people, especially those in the later stages of dementia, struggle. If your family member or friend has been known to sundown, or if she is in a more advanced stage of dementia, it is probably best to visit before lunch. She'll be more alert and likely more interested in accepting visitors.

Be aware that one visit to a parent, partner, child, or friend in a dementia care community may completely differ from another. Your family member or friend may behave differently at various times of day and even on different days of the week. A change in routine, medication, food intake, activity level, or any other potential factor can greatly alter a person with dementia's day. It's not uncommon to hear family caregivers say, "Mom wasn't like this yesterday!" This is why it is so important to remain patient throughout the caregiving experience. A great practice is to journal your times and dates of visiting. Figure out when an activity is occurring so that you can assist your family member or friend. Maybe you know that your mother loves painting, which happens on Tuesdays at 2:00 p.m. Keep track of your mother's moods during your visits, and you will probably begin to see a pattern to know the best time to see her.

Jeremy was becoming more and more aggravated as the day wore on. This was a normal occurrence for him. At about 3:00 p.m. each day, Jeremy began to pace the hallways. "Where are my mom and dad?" he would yell. Other residents would begin to get agitated, too, after hearing his cries for help.

"What is wrong with that guy?" some would ask.

Even though Jeremy was upset and looking for his parents, staff members guessed that there was probably another factor at play. Fortunately, it only took a couple of tries to solve the problem. "Hey, Jeremy, here's a snack," one said, holding out a pudding cup.

"Where are my—oh!" Jeremy stopped mid-yell, a smile crossing his face as he accepted it.

The root cause of Jeremy's sundowning was hunger. As soon as he got something to eat, Jeremy's behavior subsided. Following an episode like this, he would typically return calmly to his room and take a nap.

WAYS TO PREVENT SUNDOWNING

There are a few ways to combat sundowning—and at times, stop it altogether. Keeping a person with dementia engaged throughout the day is a great way to decrease sundowning episodes. Sometimes, boredom will make someone more agitated. That agitation, combined with normal tiredness, can result in sundowning. It is vital that all caregivers, professional and nonprofessional, in-home and community, provide interesting activities for adults with dementia throughout the day. These activities do not have to be extravagant: folding socks, reading newspapers, or even short walks around the block will provide the necessary amount of entertainment. Try to keep a person with dementia interested while not overwhelming him.

Providing regular, timed snacks will also help to combat sundowning. Jeremy was hungry. His dementia kept him from saying, "I'm feeling irritable because I'm really hungry," so caregivers had to figure that out for themselves. In many care communities, snacks are provided three times daily. When people are hydrated and full, they are much less likely to feel aggressive or irritated. Put yourself in your parent, partner, or child's shoes: How do you feel when you are tired, hungry, and overwhelmed? You probably don't act like the best version of yourself, and your loved one with dementia will not, either.

Making sure that your family member or friend with dementia has a regular schedule is another important way to combat sundowning. Keeping a person on a regular sleep-wake cycle is a great way to start the day. Imagine waking your brother with dementia, for example, at 6:00 a.m. one day, 10:00 a.m. the next, and then at 7:00 a.m. the day after that. It would throw his entire day off and mix up his internal clock. He may feel different that day but have trouble articulating that something has changed. Instead, you may just see your brother grow very irritable and frustrated for no apparent reason.

Most dementia care communities have a list of daily activities that residents can attend. Also, quiet space or breaks in the middle of a busy day are crucial for people with dementia. Letting the person have time alone for an hour—even if a caregiver is close by—can do wonders for that person's mood. A quiet, comforting space is the ideal spot for alone time. It may also be a good idea to provide the person with dementia with music of some sort.

As the clock struck 3:00 p.m. each day, Rosie would start to cry. She would wander out of her room, frustrated and depressed. She would take up her spot on the couch and lay her head in her hands.

"What's wrong?" people would ask.

"I just don't like this!" she would cry back.

It took a few weeks for the staff to realize what was upsetting Rosie so. It turned out that 3:00 p.m. was when the first shift changed for the day: the first shift left, and the second shift showed up. Numerous people moved in and out of the building at once. Rosie saw her friends—the staff—leaving and could not understand why.

After staff members caught on to this, they began hugging her before they left the building. "We'll see you tomorrow," they told her, one at a time. This was just the type of reassurance that Rosie needed. Her sundowning behavior decreased dramatically after this intervention.

The reason for Rosie's sundowning behavior became obvious after some dementia detective work on the staff's part. It could also be that Rosie used to pick up her kids from school around that time each day. When she saw people coming and going, it confused her. Rosie wondered where her children were but had trouble articulating that question. Fortunately, her trigger—the shift change—could be modified to avoid overwhelming Rosie. Although not everyone with dementia has such an obvious reason for sundowning, just a little bit of trial and error can solve some people's problems.

Sundowning, though challenging to deal with at times, is a part of dementia care. Not everyone experiences it, but many people in the later stages of dementia will get increasingly agitated and irritable as their disease progresses. Recall that it is very difficult for people with dementia to control their emotions or outbursts. A sudden stream of profanity, a physical altercation, or a drastic change in mood are just a part of dementia. Although these changes and mood swings can be upsetting, realize that a person with dementia would control her emotions better if she could. Because dementia typically affects the filter in a person's brain, she may not be able to tell you that she's tired or needs time alone. It's imperative that caregivers anticipate this need before sundowning strikes. Providing regular snacks, encouraging a normal daily routine, and providing activities while making sure to avoid overwhelming the person with dementia can all combat sundowning. These techniques and an awareness of the good times to visit someone with dementia can work wonders for your relationship.

Day Trips and Outings

"Oh, I just loved seeing those kids yesterday," Matilda exclaimed as we baked cookies with the other residents. Normally, Matilda's moderate Alzheimer's disease prevented her from holding onto new memories. In this case, however, Matilda appeared able to recall an event that had brought her a lot of joy.

Every Tuesday our group went to visit children at a local pre-school. Even though Matilda could not recall what she had done every other hour of that day, she remembered visiting the children. She remembered the special outing she had enjoyed with her fellow residents. It seemed almost as though the memory of the outing had found a special place to reside inside her brain.

Caregivers usually underestimate the importance of day trips and outings for people with dementia. This is common even in senior-living communities. Although residents in assisted-living, personal-care, and independent-living communities are often invited on community-wide outings, some residents with dementia are not offered the same opportunities. Families and friends, too, can take their loved ones with dementia on outings after picking them up from a care community. Many families, however, fear that a person with dementia will act out or behave poorly in public.

CHOOSING THE RIGHT COMMUNITY

When choosing a dementia care community for your parent, partner, adult child, or friend, it is imperative that you look for a place that invites residents on outings. Although it may seem trivial, communities that offer multiple monthly outings for residents with dementia most likely have a greater understanding and respect for their residents. It takes a proactive and dementia-friendly community to provide great outings for residents with dementia. In other words, a community that offers multiple outings probably delivers better care overall.

Diana loved going out with her fellow residents. Every time we went out for ice cream, visited the local animal shelter, or read to kids at a nearby day care, Diana was with us. "That's my seat! Don't let anybody take my front seat on the bus!" she would say, smiling as she approached the vehicle.

Outings meant a lot to Diana. Because her family did not live close by, the only day trips she went on regularly were those we did as a community. We tried to go out at least once a week, and this was a good amount of time for our residents.

When Diana's family moved her to a new community, everything changed. "I don't get out as much anymore," Diana told me sadly. Her new community didn't attempt any of the outings that we offered. In fact, it was unlikely that the residents went anywhere at all. Day after day, the residents walked the hallways and sat in the common areas. Their activity director was nowhere to be found, and there was no community bus.

Going out was important to Diana because she had been very active throughout her life. To suddenly be stuck inside all day, day after day, probably broke her heart. When searching for a dementia care community for her, Diana's family should have made sure that the community took residents on outings. Diana had grown accustomed to this, and losing the ability devastated her.

Communities should offer outings and trips for residents while being aware that these trips must be customized to suit the needs of people with dementia. For example, taking a group of residents with dementia to a museum may be challenging. Typically, residents with dementia get frustrated more easily than residents without cognitive impairments. Museums tend to involve a lot of walking, stairs, and quiet reflection. People with dementia may have trouble understanding the purpose of the trip and may quickly tire of all the walking. Although they may be able to express that they don't wish to go on the trip at all, most people with dementia lack the foresight to realize that they will not enjoy the outing. A community that attempts such an outing will likely end up with a lot of unhappy, frustrated residents soon into the excursion.

FAMILY TRIPS OUTSIDE THE COMMUNITY

When it comes to community outings, families also have the opportunity to get involved. At many communities, residents' family members can volunteer to assist with outings. If a caregiver is anxious about trying a trip with his parent, partner, or friend, for example, a trial outing with the activity director and a group of residents may be a good introduction to dementia-friendly outings. It gives someone a chance to interact with his family member or friend outside the community without the stress of doing it alone.

It was holiday time, and visitors were coming in and out of the community. Families and friends often took their loved ones out for lunch or dinner. Sometimes, family members would even take them overnight so they could enjoy holiday festivities.

Louise sat and watched as other residents were picked up. Even though her memory was very poor, she was able to understand that people around her were leaving with their families. "Hey," she said to me, pointing a wrinkled finger in my direction. I went to her side. "When is my family coming to get me?" she asked.

Residents often ask, out of the blue, about family members. This time, however, Louise's question was warranted. She could see that other residents were leaving the building, so why wasn't she going out, too? I knew that her family lived close by, so I did not know what to tell her. "I'm sure that they will be here soon," I said, touching Louise's hand softly.

"You're the sweetest," she said, smiling. "I was just wondering if they were coming to get me."

I felt sad for Louise because I neither knew where her family was nor understood why they had not come to see her. During normal weeks, I would not have worried about a resident asking about her family members—but in this case, with the holiday season underway, I wished that Louise's family would take her out for the afternoon. I sat helplessly as Louise watched quietly from the couch, a swarm of hugs and happy chatter around her.

Even if a care community does not offer many outings, families may take their family members or friends out for small trips. Make sure that you speak to staff members and sign out, if necessary, before taking a loved one out for the day—or even a few hours. Some communities encourage more outings than others do, and you'll want to make sure that your chosen community offers staff-assisted outing opportunities for its residents, too. The idea of taking a parent, partner, child, or sibling with dementia outside a community may be nerve racking at first; the following tips may help the excursion go more smoothly.

TIPS FOR OUTINGS

First, plan the trip that you will be taking with your family member or friend. Know ahead of time what types of trips she would enjoy. For example, if your mom always loved going out for lunch, try that first. Scope out a nearby restaurant ahead of time. Ensure there is enough seating and that the crowds will not be overwhelming at lunchtime. Make certain you can park close to the restaurant so that you and your mom do not have to walk too far, particularly if she has mobility issues. Once you both get inside the restaurant, are you able to sit close to a bathroom and an exit?

Be sure to adapt the outing to suit your family member or friend's needs. At the restaurant, for example, a full menu of food options could prove overwhelming to your mom with dementia. Instead of taking the menu away, modify the situation. Allow your mom to look at the menu but then take it away after a few minutes. Offer a choice of two or three food options, and let her choose from that list. Letting your mom look through the menu provides a sense of normalcy because that is the first thing most people do at restaurants. Still, you have successfully modified the trip by providing only a few meal options from which to choose.

In restaurants, especially, it is important to notify the waiter or waitress that your family member or friend has a cognitive impairment. There are a few ways to do this discreetly. As one option, you could pull the waiter aside and let him know that your mom has dementia. "My mom has dementia, but she is really excited to be here. I'm sure she would love to talk to you, but do not be alarmed if she seems a little confused," you could say. Recognize that some people are anxious about interacting with adults who have cognitive impairments, so it's important to phrase the dementia conversation with your waiter carefully. The Alzheimer's Association offers what it calls "Pardon My Companion" business cards. You can hand these cards out at restaurants or other public places where you are walking or visiting with your parent, partner, or friend in case of an incident. The cards contain brief explanations about dementia and may serve as a helpful tool when you are out and about with your family member with dementia. The cards are available online through the Alzheimer's Association (www.alz.org).[1]

Other types of outings, like trips for ice cream or a visit to a family member's home, can also be very positive. It is not recommended, however, that you take a person with dementia to her old house, even for a short period of time. Once a person with dementia has adjusted to living in a dementia care community, a trip back to her old house can be extremely confusing. She may wonder why she's visiting her old house, only to get back in the car and go home to her new location: the dementia care community. This may be acceptable for some people with dementia but it would greatly upset most dementia care community residents. A trip to another relative's house, however, may prove very pleasant.

HOLIDAYS OUTSIDE THE COMMUNITY

Over holidays in particular, picking up a parent, partner, child, or friend with dementia at his community and taking him to a holiday party can be a wonderful surprise. Recall, however, that you will need to modify this trip as well. People with dementia can easily become overwhelmed, so large parties may be challenging. Ensuring that your family member or friend has a quiet place to rest apart from the noise of the party is imperative. If you think he needs a short break from the crowd, take him into another room. It may also be useful to provide your family member or friend with a task. For example, if your aunt with dementia can still set the table, allow her to do so. She will feel like she is contributing and will probably fare better throughout the evening.

It is also important to talk to the rest of the family about how to address the person with dementia. Remind them that it's not appropriate to quiz your father with dementia about his relationship to the rest of the family. Although he may recognize some family members, others may confuse him. It is probably best, too, that the night end early for your family member with dementia. Recall that sundowning may occur, especially if your loved one is overwhelmed.

For residents with mobility issues, trips outside the community can be challenging. Some communities may let you borrow a company vehicle, or they may provide a professional caregiver to drive or drop you and your family member off at the place of your choosing.

If you are unable to take, for example, your dad on an outing, try creating a trip inside the community. Call and ask the community's director if it is okay to eat with your dad in a quiet community spot. Pick up lunch or even bring a homemade meal to enjoy with your dad in a secluded area. "Going out for lunch" doesn't mean that you need to go outside at all. For some people with dementia, doing something different and enjoying a meal with you is enough.

The ability to remain active outside the walls of a dementia care community is incredibly important for people with cognitive impairments. Many residents look forward to outings with both the community and with family members. It's understandable that the first trip with a parent, partner, child, or friend may provoke anxiety. Following a few simple guidelines can help an outing go as smoothly as possible. People with dementia deserve to live their lives in a fulfilling, engaging way that is not restricted to the inside of a building.

23

She Doesn't Recognize Me

Many people with dementia will reach a point in their disease progression when they have trouble identifying visitors who come to see them. This usually takes years and does not suddenly happen overnight. Family caregivers often express fear that their family member or friend with dementia will suddenly wake up and forget them—and this just isn't the case. Still, when a person with dementia has difficulty identifying relatives and friends, visits tend to slow down. "Mom doesn't recognize me anymore . . . why should I even come visit?" some relatives will ask. Although it can feel frustrating to continue visiting, it is imperative that families find common ground on which to connect with their loved ones.

Tabitha cruised down the hallway with her walker. We usually called her Tab, for short, and it was fitting. Tab was a petite woman with big blue eyes. Her favorite outfit was a tracksuit. She was in a moderate to advanced stage of dementia, and most of her sentences came in the form of songs. "How do you do, how, how, how, do ya do," she sang happily, tapping her walker on the floor in time to the beat. "All right, let's go," Tab whispered, trying to inspire other residents to walk somewhere with her.

Tab could often be found with a group of other residents, walking the hallway. Those who needed some guidance had Tab. Tab was not sure where she was going, but she was going somewhere—and fast. Tab's son, Mike, was often by her side. He fully embraced his mother's reality, and he recognized that she was impaired. Mike would come in the door and immediately inquire, jovially, about his mother's whereabouts. "Where is she off to today, I wonder?" he would laugh.

Once Mike located her, he would walk alongside Tab as she cruised the hallways, greeting new and old friends. He would sing and clap with her, and she would smile approvingly. One day, I met them both in the hallway. "Tab, do you want to come listen to music?" I asked. "We have a singer coming in to perform for us."

Tab's bright eyes lit up, and she turned to her son. "My husband can sing!" she said, pointing to her son. Tab nodded and kept walking, but I turned to Mike.

"Does she often think that you are her husband?" I asked, curious.

"No, not always," he replied, smiling. "Sometimes I'm my brother, sometimes I'm my dad, sometimes I'm me, and sometimes I'm someone else she knows. But always, she recognizes me. That's what is most important to me—she knows that I love her."

As Mike realized, his mother still knew him—she just could not always place him in context. She still recognized his importance to her. Although it probably pained him to realize Tab did not know exactly who he was anymore, Mike focused on the positive: Tab knew him and she knew they had a loving bond between them. That was what was most valuable to him—they still shared a positive, happy connection. What did not happen was this: She did not wake up one day and suddenly not know him. It was not a random, sudden change. Some of Tab's days were more forgetful than others, but she always knew her son.

Tab's story is not uncommon. What happens most often to people with dementia is that they have trouble placing relatives and friends in context. For example, picture yourself as a woman in your late fifties. You are visiting your father in a dementia care community, and your dad seems to know who you are, but he is having trouble identifying the relationship between you. He knows that he knows you, and he knows that you are close. He just cannot seem to figure out why he knows you so well. This is probably because of your age. When your father pictures you, he sees a young woman in her teens or twenties—or perhaps even a small child. Suddenly, you, as a grown woman, walk in the door. Because your father's ability to understand time and aging is impaired, he doesn't recognize you in context. "Who is this grown woman walking in the door?" he may think. "She sure looks like my daughter, but my daughter is just a little girl. She's here, calling me Dad, but my daughter is only 5."

CONFABULATION

It is not uncommon for those with dementia to create or make up, or *confabulate*, a relationship with a relative or friend. Confabulation happens because a person with dementia is looking to make sense of something that does not make sense to him. For example, because you are a grown woman and you look like your mother, your father may believe you are his wife. Perhaps your mother has been deceased for a few years, but your dad does not remember that anymore. You are in your fifties, and he remembers you as a child. Your dad remembers your mom as a woman in her fifties, so following that logic, you must actually be your mother. It is not that he does not know you—it is that he cannot place you on a timeline. Because people with dementia have trouble orienting to time, your dad may believe that it is still 1960. In 1960, you were just a kid. For him, these facts add up, and he confabulates a relationship with you in which you are your mother. This is why, when people with dementia look through photo albums, they often create relationships with people. Although the individuals in the photos look familiar, their exact relationship to one another is unclear to the person with dementia.

It's potentially painful when a parent does not recognize a grown child. "Why are you calling me Mom!" your mother may cry out. "I'm not your mom!" In situations like these, it may be easiest for children to call their parents by their first names as the disease progresses. "Beth, it has been great visiting with you today," you may say, addressing your own mother. It can feel awkward to address your mother this way, especially if you never referred to her by her first name, but doing so can help prevent some uncomfortable conversations.

It is crucial to remember, too, not to quiz a person with dementia about her relationships to other people. Asking "Do you remember my name?" or "Don't you remember, I'm your granddaughter!" can be unfair and unkind to a person who has trouble recalling what she had for breakfast. While your grandmother may remember that she knows you, quizzing her about your name or your exact relationship to her may not go well. Understand that she may remember you as a 5-year-old, and you no longer look like the child she once babysat.

It can be frustrating, anger inducing, and sad for relatives when their family members do not recognize them anymore. It is okay to feel this way, but it is important, too, to realize that the person with dementia is not forgetting or confusing anything on purpose. Dementia is a group of brain diseases that impair understanding, logic, and judgment.

WHILE VISITING

Penni is one of my favorite people whom I met during my time working with adults who have dementia. When her family moved her to a new community, I decided to visit her. I steeled myself, realizing that she might not remember me. As soon as she met my eyes, however, a smile beamed across her face. "It's you!" Penni cried out. "How did you find me? How did you know I was here?"

I smiled and shrugged. "I just knew where to look," I said.

As we walked down the hall, Penni introduced me to her fellow residents. "This is an old friend," she said, pointing to me. "She is just wonderful." Penni looked up at me with shining eyes.

I knew that she knew me, but she could not place me. I had never told Penni my name, even in the year that I had known her. There was no point—because of her advanced dementia, she would never have remembered my name.

"We were at that other place together, right?" Penni would ask occasionally. "We lived there," she would sometimes say upon introducing me to another resident. Penni knew me, she knew my face, she knew what I meant to her—she just could not place me in context. "I'm so glad you came to see me," she smiled, tears of joy in her eyes.

I had felt very close to Penni when she lived at my community, but I anticipated that she might not recognize exactly who I was. Because she was in a moderate stage of dementia, she was able to understand that she had known me well at some point. People in very advanced stages of dementia, however, sometimes have difficulty with even this type of recognition. Upon hearing that a loved one has dementia, many family members will ask, "When will he stop remembering who I am?" This is a complicated question that deserves a complex answer.

Unfortunately, there is no way to know for sure when or if a person with dementia will no longer recognize his loved ones. One man could spend nearly the entire course of the disease recognizing his wife, while another has trouble recognizing her even in a moderate stage of dementia. Generally, people with dementia will recognize—and be able to place—their family members late into the disease process. Your dad with dementia will not wake up one day and forget who you are. These things take time, and dementia is not sudden in course. If your dad knows you on Tuesday but seems confused about who you are on Wednesday, there is probably an underlying issue. If something like this happens, it's best to see a doctor immediately.

Events that took place years ago stay in a person with dementia's memory banks much longer than things that happened recently. Interestingly, long-term memory remains intact for nearly the entire course of the disease. This is why, if you were to visit your mother in a dementia care community, she may recognize you much faster than the care aide with whom she spends all day. Even though this care aide is familiar to her, his face and his name do not stay in her memory bank. He interacts with her nearly every day, but even so, he seems fairly new to her each time.

POINTS TO PONDER

Even if your family member or friend eventually does not seem to recognize you at all, that does not mean that she does not appreciate your visit. You are a caring, kind face and a warm hand to hold. Your presence is still needed, and you may find that she confabulates a relationship with you to fill in the missing pieces of information.

Everyone's experience with dementia is different. Some people may spend the entire course of the disease recognizing their loved ones. Typically, however, most people with dementia will have difficulty identifying relatives and friends late in the disease. This change does not happen overnight and is typically a slow, continuous loss. Being prepared for it will save a lot of heartache.

PART V

CHALLENGES AND CHANGES IN ADVANCED DEMENTIA CARE

24

The Right Approach When It Comes to Aggression

Families often struggle when a parent, partner, or sibling who has dementia begins behaving aggressively. A caregiver may say something like "My loved one never acted like this before" while another caregiver may suggest, "She will just fly off the handle at any old thing." No matter how caregivers say it, what they are referring to is the sudden, bizarre increase in aggression and agitation that someone with dementia may display.

A diagnosis of dementia may result in strong mood changes. It is important for caregivers to be aware of these changes, know how to speak to a person with dementia who is becoming aggressive, and know how to cope with the changes themselves. It is necessary to note, however, that not everyone with dementia will show signs of aggression during the course of her disease.

AGGRESSION

A person with dementia may express aggression in a physical, emotional, or even sexual way. Your spouse with dementia may yell more frequently than before. Perhaps he gets upset and agitated over small matters. Maybe he hits or slaps others for the first time. He may do or say inappropriate things at inappropriate times. This type of behavior can seem especially alarming when it is not typical for the person expressing it.

Dealing with aggression that involves a family member or friend who lives in a dementia care community can be very uncomfortable and sometimes outright upsetting. The community may call you when something happens involving your family member's care. This may leave you feeling helpless, especially since you aren't there all the time. In some situations, the director at a care community may suggest that an especially aggressive person live elsewhere. Although such suggestions or requests are rare, they do happen, especially if a resident-to-resident altercation occurs.

Mabel was aggressive in every sense of the word. She disrupted tours by calling suggestive names to the men looking for placement for their mothers and fathers, she hoarded silverware and accosted care aides, and she regularly started arguments with other residents. Fearing that this would escalate, the staff recommended that Mabel's family move her to another community. Generally, it is very difficult for care homes to request new placement for residents unless they do something egregious—and someone witnesses the event.

Mabel had dementia, but she was younger, more mobile, and much stronger than most of the other residents. Mabel also had a mood disorder, which complicated the situation. Although she could be sweet and pleasant at times, Mabel was generally quick to anger. A resident who walked in her path might get screamed at, or perhaps even pushed. Mabel's temperament wasn't good for the community, especially because she was so unlike all the other residents.

As expected, one day the worst did happen. Mabel got into a verbal altercation with another resident, and it escalated to physical violence. A care aide ran to stop the fight, but it was too late: Mabel had pushed the resident to the floor. Because the other resident was older and more fragile, she broke some bones. The woman was hospitalized, and Mabel was given a 30-day notice, which meant that her family had 30 days to find Mabel a new place to live.

People with dementia have trouble controlling their emotions because of the damage occurring in their brains. While Mabel's aggression frustrated the staff, I knew that she was not in complete control of her emotions or her reactions. I did not blame her, but I feared for her fellow residents' safety. These kinds of things are rare, but in some situations, a person with dementia does not belong in a community. Mabel's situation was not normal. She was probably a better fit for a home-care agency or perhaps a geriatric psychiatric hospital, at least for an evaluation and short stay.

When a person with dementia suddenly acts aggressive, it is because she cannot calmly express what she wishes to say or do. For example, a slap or a bite may signal that someone wants to be left alone. A sudden cry or scream may indicate that she's in pain or needs something. The part of the brain that controls a person's emotions and filter is damaged, causing an unbalanced and abnormal reaction.

HOW TO COPE

When coping with aggressive behavior, it's vital to realize that the person with dementia cannot control his reaction and is not necessarily aiming his anger at you. If your uncle with dementia calls you names or tries to slap you, it does not mean that he doesn't love you—he simply cannot fully control his emotions.

When a person with dementia first exhibits an aggressive behavior, such as verbal or physical abuse, do not just turn away. Move away from the person slowly and keep a safe distance if need be, but do your best to figure the problem out. Leaving him alone or giving him time to cool down is not necessarily the best answer. Extend your hand to him and speak calmly. Smile, try to stay positive, and do not talk in a loud voice. Be sure not to overwhelm him with a big group, either. If you were feeling upset or combative, the last thing you would want is a big group of people trying to calm you down all at once.

Of course, whenever someone is managing aggressive behavior, that person must recognize when they are in danger. For example, if your spouse is becoming more and more physically aggressive, it may not be safe for you to continue sharing a home with her. It is okay—and potentially necessary—to call the police if things escalate into a situation that you cannot control. Even though you love your spouse and she cannot control her reactions, it is imperative to keep yourself safe. You cannot successfully cope or help your family member or friend if you are in immediate danger. Again, this situation is rare. In people with dementia, aggression is usually limited in scope and does not last long.

Like most dementia-related behaviors, solving the problem means determining its root. When is your spouse becoming aggressive? What time of day is it? What is happening before she acts aggressively? Who is around? These are all important questions to ask. For example, a person who lashes out every evening may be experiencing sundowning. A different sleep cycle, a snack, or some time spent in a quiet space may solve the issue. Maybe your spouse's aggressive reaction happens whenever she comes into contact with a certain caregiver or, in the case of a care community, a particular resident. Even though Mabel's behavior was extreme, obvious triggers, such as a resident pushing her limits, would aggravate her. Mabel's behavior was traceable and had a clear cause-and-effect reaction.

YOUR APPROACH

Even though your parent, spouse, child, or friend may not have total control over her emotions, recognize that as a caregiver you can help prevent aggressive behavior. It's incredibly important to approach someone with dementia in the right way. Use these tips every time:

1. Approach from the front. Walk toward the person you are going to greet. Do not come up behind her and tap her on the shoulder. Once you are there, meet that person at eye level. For example, if your mother is in a wheelchair, crouch beside her.

2. Speak slowly and loudly enough so that the person can hear you properly. Make eye contact and smile.

3. Use the person's name and offer your hand, palm up. This will give her a chance to take your hand, instead of being touched or grabbed before she's ready.

4. Each time you approach, even if you leave for only a few minutes, repeat these same steps. You cannot be sure that a person with dementia remembers or expects you.

This type of calm, progressive approach will work wonders for lowering aggression in those with dementia and increase your chances of working with them in a positive way.

"I'm going to hit you!" Cassandra yelled. It was time for Cassandra's shower, and one of her care aides was trying to help her. Instead of offering her hand for Cassandra to hold, however, Ashley reached out to grab her. Ashley didn't mean to do it in an aggressive way, but the sudden movement and touch made Cassandra jump back.

"Hold still!" Ashley sighed, trying to use a washcloth on Cassandra's back. Cassandra reached back and swung at Ashley, nailing the right side of her face.

"Ow!" Ashley yelled. "Don't hit me!"

Ashley had told me that Cassandra was aggressive when getting a shower, but I had a feeling it had something to do with Ashley's approach—and it did. "Here, Cassandra," I said, offering my hand, palm up. Instinctively, Cassandra took it. I looked her in the eyes and smiled. "Is it okay if I help you get cleaned up?" I asked. Cassandra seemed reluctant but nodded. I let Cassandra hold the wet washcloth while I guided it over her face. She smiled as the washcloth moved gently over her forehead. "Here, hold my wrist," I suggested, letting Cassandra hold my right wrist as I washed her. Because she felt in control, Cassandra was no longer combative. Instead of being showered, she was taking a shower with help from a friend.

When Cassandra felt empowered, she did not feel the need to protect herself and therefore, lash out. Like the rest of us, people with dementia need to feel as though they have some control over what happens to them. Along the same lines, most people do not feel good when they are talked to as if they are children. Many people with dementia will respond negatively when they get talked to or about in this way—especially when it happens right in front of them.

"William, remember, you do forget things sometimes," Janice said. "Like last week, for example," she continued, despite the flames glowing in her husband's eyes, "you forgot that we had dinner plans, and then you even forgot Mary's name." She sighed. "We've known Mary for years," Janice said as a sidebar to the dementia care community's marketing manager.

Our marketing manager was trying to use Janice's feedback to assess William's cognitive state, but Janice only tore William down. William was clearly growing more and more agitated as the conversation continued. "I don't want to be in here anymore," he grumbled.

"Well, this is where we are looking at moving you now," Janice said, attempting to bring him into the conversation.

"I don't need to live anywhere except my own goddamn house!" William suddenly screamed.

Janice barely blinked an eye and turned to our marketing manager. "See," she said in a calm voice, "this is what he does. He just gets upset with me for no reason." Janice sighed, shaking her head.

Clearly, Janice's behavior influenced her husband's negative reaction. She wanted to move him to a care community because of his aggression, but she ignored the fact that her words were affecting his ability to function. Janice needed to step back and realize she was upsetting her husband. When he had gotten irritated with her in the past before his diagnosis of dementia, he was better able to control his reaction. Now, with dementia, William flew into a rage anytime his wife suggested that he had memory problems.

PAIN, DELIRIUM, AND OTHER ILLNESS

Like most of us, people with dementia may act more aggressive and irritable when they are tired, sick, or in pain. *Delirium* is a condition that comes on suddenly and is often due to other physical or mental illness. Delirium is a treatable condition, but it requires immediate medical attention because it may signal that something is wrong. For example, older adults who have urinary tract infections or have just come out of surgery are often diagnosed with delirium. When a person with dementia experiences delirium, he may suddenly become aggressive, confused, irritable, and even hallucinate. Recognize that this could be the cause of a family member or friend's aggression, especially if that aggression begins suddenly.

Pain and illness can also cause aggressive behavior in a person with dementia. Pain tends to make people irritable. But an additional diagnosis of dementia can make it hard for a person to express himself. Instead of explaining where the pain is coming from, he lashes out in anger. A caregiver who fails to pay close attention may mistake this for dementia-related aggression when the anger stems from physical pain.

In general, some amount of increased aggression is normal for people with dementia. Although it's necessary to prepare for a loved one to become more combative at some point in the disease process, it is not inevitable. Plenty of people go through the entire course of the disease without ever acting aggressively. Again, dementia is just an umbrella term for a group of diseases that cause cognitive loss over time. One person's life with dementia can differ entirely from another's, so there is no way to predict someone's experience with cognitive loss.

25

Hallucinations and Delusional Thinking

A *hallucination* is a sensation or perception that appears to be real but is not. A person can see, smell, hear, taste, or even feel a hallucination. For example, a person who hallucinates may see a dog in a room where there is no dog. The dog may appear and sound very real to the person who is hallucinating.

Hallucinations are common in some disorders, like schizophrenia. Hallucinations can also happen when people use drugs, start new medications, or even cope with a physical illness. A hallucination is not the same thing as a delusion. A *delusion* is a belief in an idea or theory that is not true. For example, a delusion common to those with dementia is that a loved one is stealing from them when that isn't the case. Delusions are more common in dementia than hallucinations, although when they do occur, hallucinations can be very alarming.

"Well aren't you just precious?" Edna asked, reaching out to touch the little boy she thought was standing next to her. But no little boy stood there. In fact, Edna wasn't standing next to anyone. Edna reached out, touched air, and smiled at us. "Could someone get him a glass of water?" she asked.

"Uhh, sure . . ." a staff member offered and went to the kitchen to fetch the "boy" something to drink. "We really need to get her checked for a urinary tract infection," the staff member whispered to me. "This is not the normal Edna I'm used to!"

As it turned out, Edna *did* have a urinary tract infection (UTI). Because the staff member knew her so well, he knew when something was wrong. He recognized that Edna was not behaving normally and decided to seek medical help immediately. Thanks to his quick action, Edna's UTI was treated with antibiotics and cleared up fairly quickly. With her UTI under control, Edna stopped hallucinating.

DEMENTIA AND HALLUCINATIONS

Many people assume that a family member or friend with dementia will hallucinate at some point. This is not true—many people with dementia do not hallucinate, especially not on a regular basis. Some types of dementia, though, such as dementia with Lewy bodies (DLB), are known for causing vivid hallucinations. People with DLB are much more likely to hallucinate than people with other forms of dementia because of the way the disease affects the brain.

Unless a doctor has told you that your family member with dementia may hallucinate, make sure that she has a full medical checkup after an episode of hallucinating. In most cases, when a person begins hallucinating, the caregiver should seek medical help quickly. Often, as with Edna's UTI, a hallucination signals an underlying medical issue. It is imperative that a caregiver doesn't write off hallucinations as a normal part of dementia. They are not necessarily normal for everyone.

No matter what, it's important to avoid alarming your loved one when she hallucinates. As in all situations regarding dementia care, it is imperative that you "play along" with what she is seeing. For example, if she sees a neighbor in the garden who does not exist, be sure to agree that you also see the neighbor. This goes back to the idea of embracing your loved one's reality. Recall that what she's experiencing is very real for her.

Hallucinations can sometimes frighten both the person with dementia and the caregiver. In some cases, hallucinations will make it hard for people with dementia to live their lives. They may be afraid to sleep, eat, or walk around the house. Many stories are told about hallucinations making it difficult for people with dementia to get enough sleep. Some people will hallucinate that bugs or animals are in their bed at night, while others may decide that people walk in and out of their rooms. Although it is challenging, caregivers must decide to face the problem directly. Arguing with a person who has dementia about the hallucination or trying to convince her that the hallucination isn't real will not prove effective. Hallucinations are extremely real to those experiencing them.

"What are they doing out there?" Melody asked, eyes wide. Her husband, Bill, peered out the kitchen window.

"What is who doing out where?" he asked, squinting into the dark night at the trees near the border of their property line.

"Those people," Melody said, pointing. "Look at them. They are all standing around in the trees!"

Suddenly frightened and confused, Bill looked harder. "I don't see anything!" he replied. "Let me go get a flashlight."

"No, no." Melody shook her head. "I don't know what they are up to. It looks like they are just standing around. Maybe they will go away soon."

Over the course of a couple of weeks, Bill realized that Melody was seeing people who were not there. Every night they would argue about the presence of people in the trees outside, and every night Melody would insist that they were there.

Bill did not go along with Melody's story, and this strained their relationship. He eventually moved her into a long-term-care community because he could not cope with her odd behaviors. Melody had DLB, which explained her ongoing hallucinations. Bill had difficulty accepting that Melody's dementia affected her perception of the world around her. She did not create these stories to scare her or her husband—truly, she saw, and believed she saw, people outside their window.

VISUAL CONFUSION

"There he is," Terrence said, pointing at the mirror. "That's my neighbor, Ben."

Terrence's son, taken aback, watched as his father talked to the mirror.

"Hey, Ben, what's going on?" Terrence jovially asked the mirror. Terrence went on to describe how his day had been and offered to meet Ben outside their rooms for dinner. "I'll see you in a few minutes," Terrence told the mirror.

Terrence and his son walked out of the room and waited for Ben. "I'm not sure where Ben is," Terrence said, looking up and down the hallway.

Afraid of what would happen if his father waited too long, Terrence's son spoke up. "Dad, let's just head down to dinner, and I'm sure that Ben will meet us there," he said.

Terrence shrugged. "I guess so!" he agreed.

Thankfully, Terrence's son decided to embrace his father's reality. Terrence's brain was unable to make sense of his own reflection. He could not understand why and how he had aged so much because the man he remembered being was not that old. It made sense, then, why Terrence believed that his aged reflection was a neighbor. He created an identity for Ben and even gave him a name. Note that although bizarre, this is not so much a hallucination as a mix-up. Terrence's reflection existed, but he gave it a different identity. Sometimes, a person with dementia will behave as though he is hallucinating even if he is not truly experiencing a hallucination. A person may confuse objects, light, noise, or other items in his environment for something else. For example, a large chair in the corner of a room could look like a big, hulking bear to a person with dementia.

Beth stood in the hallway and pointed, her eyes growing wide. "Look at that!" she cried out, tugging at my sleeve. "Look at those leaves falling inside."

I looked down the hall, but I didn't see any leaves. Thinking that she was hallucinating, I probed further. "Where are the leaves coming from?" I asked.

"Right there," she answered and pointed to another resident. I looked and then realized that the other resident wore a shirt covered with a pattern of falling, brightly colored leaves.

Because the other resident was walking away from Beth, it looked to Beth like the leaves were moving. This was not a hallucination but a moment of confusion in Beth's mind. Dementia is a brain disease, compromising Beth's vision, perception, and spatial awareness. If Beth had seen leaves falling but the resident with the leaf-patterned shirt didn't exist, she would have been hallucinating. In this particular instance, however, Beth was unable to distinguish between a shirt with a design of leaves on it and real leaves.

It's important to know when people with dementia are truly hallucinating and when they are confusing stimuli in their environment. For example, maybe a strained light coming through a foggy window makes it look as if another person is in the room. Perhaps a dark shadow on the floor or a black rug looks like a hole. When a person with dementia seems to be hallucinating, it is crucial to determine the cause.

HOW TO COPE

A helpful tip is to record when and where your loved one with dementia perceives a potential hallucination. What is he seeing, hearing, smelling, tasting, or feeling? In what room does this happen and at what time of day? Did this hallucination begin suddenly, or has it been around for a long time? Once you know where the hallucination comes from, you are better equipped to deal with it. If something in the environment is the culprit, change it. In the case of the foggy window, perhaps drawing the shades would keep the room from looking as though another person was present. In the case of the black rug, removing it from the room would probably eliminate your family member or friend's fear of falling through a hole in the floor.

The above examples show how making changes to the environment can help your parent, partner, child, or friend avoid any confusion over what he is seeing. At other times, however, you may need to take him to a doctor to check for an underlying medical condition or a reaction to medication. In any event, it's important to understand that hallucinations are sometimes a part of the disease process. Whether the hallucination is pleasant or unpleasant, caregivers must find a way to cope. It is always essential to embrace a person with dementia's reality, even when that reality seems far fetched.

26

Aphasia, Second Languages, and Word Salads

For many families, visiting a parent, partner, child, sibling, or friend in dementia care becomes an important part of a regular routine. When someone with dementia has trouble speaking, however, many people begin to question whether they should visit at all. Because dementia is a group of brain diseases, it has an impact on much more than just memory and perception—it also affects a person's ability to communicate.

People with dementia will have difficulty speaking, writing, and understanding as the disease progresses. As a caregiver, you will likely find it more and more challenging to understand what a person with dementia is trying to express. Caregivers need to learn to observe body language, understand facial cues, and watch for hand gestures as their family member or friend slowly loses the ability to communicate properly.

Dementia is an umbrella term that affects everyone differently, so there is no way to predict the entire course of a person's experience with the disease. While some people will be able to communicate well throughout their life with dementia, others will mix up words, jumble phrases, or even rely on a few key terms to express themselves. Some may lose the ability to speak entirely, even early in the disease, when it seems as though their other faculties are intact. The term for this is *aphasia*, a language disorder, or group of disorders, that affects a person's ability to understand and express thoughts and ideas.

WORD SALADS

"What did you do earlier today?" Pam asked her mother.

"We went fish to the mall red," Patty answered.

Pam opened her mouth to respond but then closed it again. She did not understand what her mother had said.

"You did what?" she asked again.

"We went right to the mall after lunch," Patty responded, tilting her head to the side. "That's what I said the first time, wasn't it?"

Pam realized that something was wrong with her mother's speech. Sometimes, everything would make sense, and other times, it was as though Patty's sentences were a mix of words. It appeared, too, as though Patty was quite sure she was always saying what she meant to say.

"What book is the house on?" she asked, pointing to the clock in the other room. Her tone was normal and her voice was calm, but the words she spoke did not work together.

This type of speech is sometimes referred to as a *word salad*. While professionals don't use this term, it perfectly describes the way some people with language disorders speak. A word salad is exactly what it sounds like: a mix of words that make sense independently but have been thrown together in a sentence that does not mean anything. Sometimes, people with dementia use word salads when attempting to communicate. When this happens, it's best if caregivers try to fill the confusing blanks with information that makes sense. For example, if Patty had been walking in the mall and had pointed to the restroom and said, "Do you need dinner together now?" she might be asking her companion to join her in the women's restroom.

Recognizing these uncontrollable communication problems in yourself is likely uncomfortable and distressing for people with dementia. Therefore, as with other areas of dementia caregiving, it is best to ignore the mistake and continue the conversation as normally as possible. Use other clues to figure out what the person is saying. Suggesting something like "You aren't making any sense" will not help you or your family member or friend. Recall that she cannot help what is happening and is doing her best to communicate with you.

SECOND LANGUAGES

As dementia progresses, people who have learned other languages tend to lose the ability to speak them. Often, adults with dementia will forget languages that are not their native tongue.

Silvia turned to her table partner and friend, Emma. "Can you pass me the salt?" she asked. Emma nodded and handed it to her.

"Gracias, mi amor. ¿Tú quieres más agua?" Silvia asked her friend.

"What!" Emma cried out. "What did you just say?"

"What do you mean, what did I say?" Silvia asked, startled, in her Cuban accent. "I asked if you wanted more water. What did you think I said?"

Silvia's first language was Spanish, and she was clearly beginning to transition back to speaking only Spanish. Every so often, Silvia would answer a question, say a word, or speak a sentence entirely in Spanish. She did not realize that she was not speaking the same language as everyone else around her, either. Emma often got irritated and confused when this happened, but Silvia would continue speaking as though nothing had happened.

"I don't know what she's talking about," Emma announced one day at dinner. "She's not speaking English, I don't think."

"I know English!" Silvia cried out. "I've been living here since I was three years old! Dios mio!"

Because language is learned over time, it gets stored in our long-term memory. Even though dementia eats away at a person's short-term memory first, it also eventually impairs a person's long-term memory later in the course of the disease. For people who speak a second language, this can be a real problem. Many adults with dementia will begin to lose their ability to speak their second language over time. What tends to stick around the longest is a combination of two languages and then, finally, only the first language. This can cause serious issues when caregivers don't speak the same language as their family member or friend.

"I don't get it," Brian said. "He used to speak perfect English!"

Brian's uncle, Gabriel, was originally from Czechoslovakia. He was very hard to understand, especially because his sentences moved fluently from one language to another. Although he used to speak fluent English, Gabriel now held only a few key phrases. "I love you," he would tell caregivers or ask, "Oh, yeah?" when he thought someone spoke to him. He knew how to say yes, no, and a few other words, too.

Generally, however, it was unclear whether Gabriel actually understood what was said to him. Sometimes, it seemed as though he understood English but could not speak it. Other times, it seemed as though Gabriel had no idea what anyone around him was saying.

Language loss can be challenging for many families, particularly when a person moves from one language to another. Again, the best thing a caregiver can do in this situation is to rely on the person's other cues. Is he pointing or gesturing to something? Does he look sad or happy? Using context clues can help caregivers deduce what someone with dementia is trying to communicate, even if the words make no sense.

CURSING

"My mother never used to speak like this," Caitlin said, shaking her head. "I'm so sorry."

"Shut the hell up, bitch!" Caitlin's mother, Bev, yelled at a caregiver, paying no heed to her daughter's embarrassment. Bev was normally a very sweet woman, but when she got upset she used some rough language. Bev cursed, yelled, and even threw racial slurs at some of her caregivers. "I don't want a shower! I'm perfectly clean!" she yelled at an approaching aide. "I don't need your goddamn nasty hands all over me!"

It's not uncommon for people with dementia to lose their social filter, which prevents them from saying inappropriate things, as the disease progresses. When young, we're usually taught to think before speaking. But a person with dementia may have difficulty holding back some of her immediate thoughts. The part of her brain that controls automatic language—the frontal lobe—can become damaged in some types of dementia. For example, when a woman without dementia thinks, "I don't want any help from this obnoxious person," she may keep it to herself because she has learned not to be rude. That same woman, if she has dementia, may have lost the filter that tells her to keep silent and say, "I don't want any help from you. You are obnoxious, and you can go straight to hell!"

When the filter is impaired, so is a person's ability to hold back racial slurs, inappropriate sexual advances, and vulgar language. Bev had never spoken like that before, but her brain had always known those bad words. She had learned, over time, to avoid saying mean or nasty things to people. Because dementia had ruined her filter, though, Bev said exactly what she thought, exactly when she thought it.

This can be embarrassing for family caregivers. They need to remember, however, that dementia is a brain disease that impairs the way a person speaks and thinks. Loved ones with dementia do not mean to say the awful things that sometimes come out of their mouths. They just lack complete control over their own language.

PHRASE REPETITION

Sometimes, people in more advanced stages of dementia use one phrase as their main way to communicate. For example, caregivers may notice that their parent, partner, child, or friend has become fixated on or obsessed with a few words or a couple of different sayings. Often, these phrases do not make complete sense in context.

"Oh, lookie here, look, look at that," Laura said. "See that thing?" she motioned, pointing to a table in the other room.

Laura was in an advanced stage of Alzheimer's disease. She was very pleasant, very kind, and often took up post sitting on a couch in her dementia care community's hallway. Laura loved talking to people who sat beside her or walked by, but her phrases tended to be the same—and they tended not to make sense in context. Her most often-used phrases centered around the idea of "look at that."

"Look at that. You've got—one, two, three, four, five," she said, counting a caregiver's fingers while holding her hand. "Oh, lookie here, somebody else is coming down, down here." She smiled, acknowledging a visitor walking by her couch.

Because of her dementia, Laura's brain made it difficult for her to find other words to say what she wanted to express. For one reason or another, her brain focused on the word "look." Even though Laura used the same phrase all the time, in her mind, she may have been thinking or speaking about very different things. One "look at that" could be her version of saying, "I really like seeing you," while another could be, "I'm getting hungry." In context, the phrase "look at that" did not always make sense, but Laura's meaning behind the words changed to fit her needs and mood. It became up to the caregiver to decipher exactly what Laura needed.

"I want to die, I want to die, I want to die, die, die," Becky cried out. Becky was also in an advanced stage of dementia, like Laura. Unlike Laura, however, Becky's repetition was more disturbing and dark. Dementia affects different people in different ways, and for Becky, her common phrase "I want to die" showed how uncomfortable she was. Becky was often in pain due to another physical condition.

Sometimes, Becky would offer up other words or phrases. Typically, though, it was just, "I want to die." This disturbed a lot of visitors who came to the community. Even if Becky was not upset, many of her phrases suggested otherwise. Death, dying, and crying out for her mother were all typical in Becky's vernacular.

People in later stages of dementia will sometimes get "stuck" on a phrase or two and use it repeatedly. It's important to remember that dementia affects the way a person's brain stores and retrieves information. Although she may want to say something different, a person with dementia may have trouble expressing herself. Sometimes, even in the quiet dining room, Becky would randomly call out, "Momma, Momma, Momma!" It was not a cry for her mother, really, but it was a cry for assistance. Becky was hungry and needed help using her utensils. "Momma, Momma, Momma" became a way for Becky to express her needs and wants. Even though she would have preferred to say, "I'm hungry. Please bring me a fork," Becky's brain only allowed her to retrieve a few odd phrases to communicate.

COMPLETE LOSS

Some people with dementia experience a complete loss of language. Typically, right at the end of the disease, most people lose the ability to speak at all. Some, however, lose it much sooner.

Kevin was very expressive, even though he did not speak. Every once in a while, Kevin would utter a word or phrase, but generally he was silent. Even when he laughed, Kevin mimed laughing. Sounds of laughter would not come out of his mouth. Instead, Kevin would slap his knee and open his mouth as though he were audibly laughing. It was clear from his motions that he was enjoying himself, even though he could not communicate using words or sounds.

"I don't know why I bother coming to visit," Kevin's daughter, Cindy, said one day. "Dad can't understand what I'm saying, and he never talks back."

Cindy was standing right next to her father as she spoke these words. Frustrated that she would say this in front of him, I tried to include Kevin in the conversation.

"I'm sure you're glad when your daughter comes to visit," I said to Kevin, smiling. Kevin did a little dance and touched his daughter's arm.

Kevin's daughter assumed that Kevin did not understand what was going on around him because he could not speak. Although occasionally Kevin couldn't respond to cues or completely understand his relationship with the world around him, at other times Kevin knew exactly what was said to him. Clearly, he knew his daughter and appreciated her visits.

COPING

Even if a family member or friend cannot speak or doesn't seem to understand, it is imperative that caregivers do not talk about the person in front of him. It is also important for caregivers to include their parent, partner, or friend in the conversation and continue to visit even when he cannot express himself. The ability to use context clues and body language is incredibly helpful when talking to a person who has aphasia. Recognize that the words a person with dementia speaks may not match what he actually feels. It's up to you, as a caregiver, to decipher what he means.

27

Dietary Changes

Food is a huge part of most people's lives and often a hobby as well. Many adults take pleasure in trying new types of food, cooking, and baking. Unfortunately, dementia can affect the way someone enjoys and experiences food. A person's ability to taste certain things, chew certain foods, or even swallow becomes affected as dementia progresses. Typically, in the latest stages of dementia, a person will struggle to ingest food at all. Families need to be prepared to handle the dietary changes that come with a person's cognitive loss.

Jess sat at the table, eating a sandwich that her daughter had brought. The sandwich looked delicious, but Jess seemed to be struggling. The thick bread and the meat inside proved difficult for her to chew. Still, Jess's daughter insisted that she knew her mother's needs. "Mom never eats enough," Julie complained. "That's why she's losing so much weight! Look at how rail thin she is."

Jess was too thin, but Julie ignored a potential issue regarding her mother's food intake—that she could not eat some of the things put in front of her. Still, Julie protested that Jess was choosing to eat too little. "That's why she's here," Julie said, holding up her hands for emphasis. "She needs the staff to push food and liquids on her."

Julie did not understand that her mother had lost weight partly because she could not easily eat certain foods. The family was doing what they thought was right—putting plenty of food in front of her—but it was the wrong type of food. Jess needed to be on a "mechanical soft" diet, eating foods that are soft and easy to chew. Grinding tough foods, such as meat, was another option. Because Jess had dementia, she couldn't express her trouble eating. She might not have understood why she was not able to eat the food her family gave her.

When a person with dementia moves into a care community, a nurse, doctor, or even a speech therapist will assess her diet. This professional may recommend that a person with dementia follow a diet different from her current one. For some residents, this may include food items that are easy to pick up, such as sandwiches or other finger foods. Some residents may be on a "puree" diet and only eat foods that have been pureed. Residents who are in advanced stages of dementia typically have difficulty feeding themselves or swallowing. They may require a diet that helps prevent choking during mealtimes. Some families find these changes difficult to accept, but altering diets allows residents to safely get the right amount of nutrition.

Some family members and friends of residents in dementia care have trouble understanding what their loved ones can and cannot eat. This becomes especially true during the holidays.

Kara had always loved chocolate, which her son remembered. As Kara's dementia progressed, however, she could no longer feed herself or eat the same foods. She was a huge risk for choking, so her diet had been changed to puree. Kara's son lived in another country, though, and he did not see his mother often or keep in contact with his siblings.

Kara's birthday was approaching, and her son sent her a box of chocolates in the mail. "Happy Birthday, Mom!" the card read. I sat and stared at the box of chocolates. I had no idea how to get hold of Kara's son, especially because the other siblings were not in contact with him. I was sad for Kara, even if she had no idea what was happening. I knew she could not enjoy the chocolates, at least not in this form.

Suddenly realizing there was another option, I contacted our chef. "Can you puree this down for me?" I asked.

"Sure," she said. "I'll add some whipped cream so it's not just pure chocolate. Bring me the box and I'll get that together for you." Our chef pureed the box of chocolates with some whipped cream and a little bit of milk. I took the candied mix up to Kara. With some help from the staff, she was able to enjoy her birthday gift.

Kara was fortunate because our chef was able to puree her box of chocolates. This, of course, is not always going to be an option for a dementia community. To avoid these circumstances, review your family member or friend's diet with her care providers to determine what types of gifts or treats are appropriate. This will ensure she's able to enjoy your gift safely. It is important for families to respect residents' diets in dementia care communities. An accidental dietary mishap can be fatal to a person who has trouble swallowing. Although you may like the idea of giving your dad with dementia cheese cubes to snack on, they may be too chewy for him to handle. If you still choose to bring him cheese cubes and they are not in his diet plan, there is no recourse you can take if something bad happens.

UTENSIL USE

Hillary was always up and about. It was difficult for her to sit and enjoy a meal with her tablemates because she was so distractible. Often, Hillary did not like to sit down for long periods of time. She was also not able to feed herself using any utensils. She could often be seen picking up a fork, looking at it, and putting it down again. She would usually put her utensils next to other people's plates because she wasn't sure of their purpose. Still, Hillary was not at the point where she wanted or needed a staff member to feed her.

Knowing this, the doctor recommended a "finger food" diet for Hillary. When the community had chicken breast, the staff gave it to Hillary on a bun. When the community had soup, they put it in a mug for her to drink. Hillary got to enjoy the same foods as her fellow residents, but she was able to do so in her own way.

Eating utensils had become a real challenge for Hillary. Although eating on her modified diet was not as clean and tidy as using a knife and fork, Hillary was able to maintain her independence and still feed herself. Hillary's diet also allowed her to get up and move around, taking the food with her. Her nutrition wasn't at risk because she was able to get the right amount of nutrition in the right way.

Many people, especially in the later stages of dementia, will lose their ability to eat as cleanly as Hillary. Some people may be on soft food diets but, wanting to feed themselves, choose to continue eating with their hands. In situations like these, a *plate guard* is a good option. A plate guard is an object that curves around a plate and prevents food from falling off the edge of the plate. While this can be messy and look unpleasant, recognize that it is an important way for a person with dementia to remain independent. No one is feeding her. Instead, she's in control of what and when to eat.

In some instances, helping a person with dementia take a few bites of food may then "cue" him to continue the process. For example, some people with dementia will be able to continue eating with a fork once a caregiver helps them put food on the fork. If your dad has trouble using a fork, you may choose to put your hand under his hand and guide the fork to his mouth. After a few tries, your dad may be able to do the motion on his own. For many people with dementia, the skill of eating by oneself is not completely lost until very late in the disease process. Some people just need a little bit of help to get started with eating a meal.

Late in the disease, people with dementia will lose the ability to feed themselves at all. No amount of cueing or reminding can help a person who has forgotten how to take food in. In situations like these, it is imperative that a caregiver feed that person his entire meal. In dementia care communities, professional caregivers know who needs assistance with feeding. They help residents with eating and drinking throughout the course of a mealtime. Caregivers are encouraged to help residents with dementia feel empowered while eating. For example, the person with dementia can hold onto a caregiver's feeding hand or wrist while the caregiver holds the utensil. This allows the person to feel as though he is still involved in the feeding process—it is not happening *to* him but *with* him.

NOT EATING

Some people with dementia will stop eating or will begin eating only certain foods. When this happens, find a solution by becoming a dementia detective. Many people with dementia will begin craving sweets at some point in the disease process. Although this seems odd, it is because, as dementia progresses, a person loses the ability to distinguish between tastes. Sweet foods may become more attractive to people with dementia, even if they didn't indulge in sweets earlier in life.

Encouraging a family member or friend with dementia to eat more can include a number of approaches. Ensure that she is eating in a well-lit environment. Make certain that distractions in the area, such as overly stimulating music or excess people, are limited. This can help your loved one eat more food. Recognize that when it comes to eating and dementia, people's needs change, and they may approach food differently. For example, people who were once big eaters may progress in their dementia and lose the ability to eat or enjoy eating as much as they used to.

BEING PREPARED

Caregivers should be aware that how well their parent, partner, child, or friend who has dementia can enjoy and eat certain foods, or even feed himself, is going to change. A doctor or other medical practitioner can advise a family on the best type of diet for their loved one. Respecting his dietary needs is an important part of providing him with the best possible life after a diagnosis of dementia. Things will not be how they used to be, but you can still have a beautiful and enjoyable time with your family member or friend if you just adjust your expectations.

28

Caregiver Stress and Cultivating Patience

"Patience is a virtue, possess it if you can. Always found in woman, but never found in man."

A 92-YEAR-OLD DEMENTIA COMMUNITY RESIDENT

Patience is, without a doubt, a virtue. When it comes to dementia care, caregivers may find it very challenging to remain patient. People with dementia ask the same questions again and again. They have bathroom-related accidents, falls, and sometimes create messes while eating. They follow caregivers around, trying to find something productive to do. People with dementia will try a person's patience on a regular basis. It is sometimes a feat of strength to stay kind, calm, and easygoing in the face of all these trials.

The most important thing to remember is that people with dementia don't intend to get on anyone's nerves. They do not want to repeat questions, they do not want to have accidents, and they do not wish to be a burden—but that is how this disease operates. It is not their fault when their behavior is irritating. People with dementia no longer have the cognitive control they once had. The things they like may be different. The way they walk and talk may change. But they are still human beings with feelings, and it is imperative to treat them as such.

Although it is frustrating to hear the same question multiple times, it is important to continue providing responses in a pleasant way. Because his short-term memory is so damaged, a person with dementia does not realize that he has previously asked the same question.

"What time is it?" Dave asked.

"It is three o'clock in the afternoon," I replied with a smile.

"Okay, thank you," he said. Two minutes later, he asked again. "Hey, what time is it?"

"It's around three o'clock in the afternoon," I replied with a smile. Another two or three minutes passed, and Dave called out for me. "Hey! What time of day is it?"

I sighed quietly to myself and closed my eyes. I took a moment to breathe before answering.

"It is three o'clock in the afternoon," I answered, walking over and touching his hand.

"Oh, thank you, you are the sweetest!" he said, smiling.

I left the room because I knew I needed a break from the questions. Dave was a kind soul who did not deserve for me to lose my patience. I could feel myself beginning to get frustrated, and I didn't want to take that out on him. In Dave's mind, he had only asked the question once. He had no idea that he had already asked the same question three times within a few minutes.

Many people say to me, "Wow, you must be really patient to work with people who have dementia!" Although I have a lot of patience for people with dementia, I am not without my breaking point—and no caregiver is. Instead of feeling guilty that my patience is not flawless, I take time apart from my residents in order to give them the absolute best part of myself. This is a technique I recommend to every caregiver. It is imperative to know your breaking point and take time to separate yourself from the person you are caring for.

Your loved one with dementia deserves your best. If your brother with dementia constantly asks questions, don't lose sight of the fact that he is not doing it to frustrate you. Keep that in mind and take a break. Leave the room for a while. Take a few deep breaths and clear your mind. Recuperate, take a few minutes to regain your positive energy, and return to your brother. Lashing out at him for asking the same question for the sixth time is not going to solve any problems; instead, he will just wonder why you are so angry and assume it is because you don't like him. People with dementia are incredibly intuitive and often focus on another person's emotions.

"Mom! I told you before, we are going to the store," Jeff hissed at his mother, Belinda. "If you would just wait and see where we are going, you could stop asking about it." Belinda had dementia, and her constant stream of questions frustrated Jeff to no end. Belinda was upset. She did not understand why her son was so cruel to her. In Belinda's mind, she had only asked about their destination once.

Five minutes passed, and Belinda asked again. "Honey, where are we going?" This time, instead of answering, Jeff sulked in angry silence. He did not want to answer his mother. "Jeff, where are we going?" Belinda asked loudly, thinking he must not have heard her.

"Mom! We are going to the store!" Jeff yelled. "The store. We are going to the store."

Belinda's eyes filled with tears. How had she raised such an angry man? She hoped that he did not speak to his wife this way.

Over time, Jeff ruined his relationship with his mother. "I don't understand why my son is so angry with me all of the time," Belinda would tell other people. She could not remember what triggered Jeff's anger, but she knew it happened when she was around. She assumed it was because she had been a bad mother. Even though Belinda forgot what time of day it was, what she had eaten for breakfast, and where they were going that day, she never forgot how her son treated her. Belinda spent the rest of her life believing that her son hated her.

Even though a family member or friend with dementia may not recall what you said, she will remember how you said it. Positive energy goes a very long way in dementia care. Answering a question with kindness and patience is imperative, even if you feel as though you have no energy left. As a caregiver, you will become frustrated at times. It is okay to get frustrated—as long as the person you are caring for doesn't see you that way.

There will be days when you feel as though you cannot carry on. This is when it is important to seek respite care, an in-home-care agency, or perhaps even a long-term dementia care community. Dementia care can be incredibly exhausting, but it is important that a person with dementia never realizes that she affects you in this manner. No one wants to feel as though she is exhausting to spend time with. No one wants to feel like a burden.

SEEKING RESPITE CARE

Before you lose your cool or say something you regret to your parent, partner, child, or friend, look into respite care. Even if you feel it is not time for a dementia care community, it may be time to seek some extra help. Many dementia care communities offer respite stays. A respite stay means that a person can stay for a limited time in a community and receive all the benefits of being a full-time resident. Many respite-stay residents will stay in communities for 10, 15, or even 30 days at a time, day and night. Families are expected to complete the same paperwork and information that long-term-care residents' families do. They should also receive the same orientation that new residents' family members receive.

Typically, families seek respite care because they need a break, are going on vacation, or are trying to decide if a dementia community is the right choice for their family member. A respite stay may give a family the information they need to decide about long-term care, but it is not advisable to "try out" a number of communities in a row in this fashion. People with dementia typically have trouble adjusting to new environments, so multiple moves in quick succession can be very upsetting for them.

HOSPICE AND PALLIATIVE CARE

When most people hear the word "hospice," they cringe with fear. Traditionally, hospice has been for people within six months of death. But people use hospice and palliative care for many other things. For example, a hospice organization could care for a person with dementia who has a wound that doesn't heal. This is what the "palliative care" part of hospice is for: providing relief from physical pain or even mental stress.

Dementia care communities, and assisted-living or personal-care communities for that matter, use hospice companies frequently. It is not uncommon to see a couple of different hospice organizations in a care community. Different residents will use different hospice organizations depending on their care needs. Usually, hospice companies will provide showers to their patients, even though the care aides at the community can help with resident showers, too. Many hospice companies will also cover the cost of adult briefs, wound care products, and other incontinence supplies. Some hospice organizations go to care communities to provide education about their services, and they will often host a bingo game, provide snacks, or even bring in pets for pet therapy while there.

Hospice is a fantastic resource for many families. Even if your family member or friend does not appear "ready" for hospice care, it could be worth asking an administrator at the care community for more information. Hospice organizations are nearly always accepting new patients, and many companies will come in to assess residents for free.

COPING WITH CAREGIVER STRESS

Caregivers bear an incredible amount of weight on their shoulders. They have their own lives to worry about on top of caring for another person. Whether it is at home or in a dementia care community, caring for someone with dementia can take a toll on a person.

Fortunately, there are ways to combat and cope with the stress of caregiving.

Caregivers must make time for themselves. Many people feel guilty if they are not entirely devoted to providing hands-on care, but they are being unfair to themselves. Being a perfect caregiver does not mean devoting yourself 24 hours a day, seven days a week to your parent, partner, child, or friend's care. It means that you can ensure that she is safe and comfortable even if you are not by her side. This may mean bringing in a home-care agency, choosing a dementia care community, using an adult day-care center, or seeking another option.

One of the benefits of choosing a dementia care community is that caregivers are able to provide their family member or friend with 24-hour care without having to be at the person's side. Staff members take care of the person's physical and emotional needs, but caregivers are able to visit as frequently as they want. Many people find that they are able to provide more positive emotional energy for their loved one with dementia when they do not have to handle the physical caregiving.

Tim had been putting his mother's care first for three years. He had turned down nearly every invitation to go out: birthday parties, dinner dates, yoga class. In turn, Tim was miserable, but he didn't really think about how unhappy he actually was. Tim accepted that this was his life and that his job was to care for his mother, Mary, no matter how much care she needed. Mary had cared for Tim when he was growing up. Now, Tim believed that it was his turn to do the caregiving—all of it.

Tim's marriage suffered. His health suffered. His friendships suffered. Even his children, grown and out of college, did not hear from him much, unless it was an update about Grandmother's dementia. Still, Tim shouldered the weight of the caregiving, with no help from anyone else—including his own sister. Tim's sister lived in another city, and somehow Tim had become the sole caregiver. Tim was unwilling to invite a home-care agency into his house or take his mother to a dementia care community.

When Tim's mother passed away, Tim was stricken with sadness, as anyone would be. He could not ignore, however, the small amount of relief he felt. Even though Tim felt terrible for admitting it, he was relieved that he could finally return to a normal life. What Tim did not expect, however, was the time that it took to piece together a normal existence.

He had given up many nights out and a number of phone calls with other friends and family. Although it had been worth it to care for his mother, Tim wished that he had done a better job of managing his time. Perhaps if he had taken a little more time for himself during the caregiving process, he would have been less stressed and more able to maintain relationships with people other than his mother.

The weight of caring for another person can be crushing. For Tim, the caregiving burden took the majority of his time and energy. If Tim had been able to seek help in the form of other caregivers, respite stays, or long-term-care options, perhaps he would have been better able to care for himself, too.

Taking time to exercise, eat sensibly, and be social are all important parts of staying healthy when caregiving. It is not uncommon to hear caregivers say things like "But I don't have time to exercise," or "I don't have time to go out with my friends." Enjoying your life and making time for things that you love will make you a better caregiver. Staying at your family member or friend's bedside and avoiding contact with the outside world will most likely cause you to harbor some resentment toward your loved one.

The ability to accept caregiving assistance from outside sources can also provide you with more emotional resources. Taking advantage of respite care, dementia care communities, or other help can give you the strength to be a great caregiver. When caregiving is not the most important piece of your life, you have more room to live. This can make caring for another person much, much easier.

29

Preserving Hope

I wrote this book to provide insight into dementia care communities: the differences among them, the services they provide, who lives there, who works there, and, most of all, how you can make the most of such a community for your friend or family member. You now have an idea of what to expect when moving your parent, partner, sibling, adult child, or friend into long-term care. But above all else, I hope this book has eased your mind about this decision. The choice to move someone into a dementia care community is challenging. You will have your doubts, your concerns, and even arguments with yourself and others. Still, you have a reason to hope for the best. You are making a decision that affects both you and your family member, but it can be a beautiful choice.

Perhaps you are the designated power of attorney and have decided to move your mother with dementia into a care community. Maybe other members of your family disagree with your choice: They wish to care for her at home. They don't believe that long-term-care communities are the best option, especially based on what they've heard about them. It is important to trust yourself as the power of attorney to make the best, healthiest choice for you and your mother. There will always be naysayers. In some cases, siblings battle for years over the idea that one of them has chosen to move Mom or Dad into long-term care. It is not a crime to make the best decision for a person with dementia, especially when that person cannot decide for herself.

It may be helpful, if possible, to get a person in the earliest stages of dementia to let you know where she'd like to live as her dementia progresses. Recognize, however, that a person with very advanced dementia may not be able to live at home any longer, even if that is where she wants to stay.

Dementia care communities exist to provide caregivers with another option. They represent an opportunity to give your family member or friend a better life than she could receive at home. This isn't to say that you would not provide the best care possible but instead to suggest that care communities are equipped with all the tools necessary to provide 24-hour physical and emotional care to adults with dementia. Dementia care communities preserve and draw out the things that your family member or friend with dementia still possesses: the ability to love, learn, and be excited about life. Many families are concerned that they are "caging" a loved one. Think, instead, that a community where people with dementia can be safe and secure from the outside world may not be such a terrible thing. They are in a place with adults their own age and cognitive level and have the opportunity to make true friendships.

Perhaps you felt uncomfortable learning that some people with dementia will have romantic relationships with others in the community. Although that can be unsettling to think about, consider that those with dementia deserve the opportunity to meet and engage with new people. They deserve the chance to make friends, create relationships, and even have a romantic partner if they so choose. A dementia care community allows for this in a way that home care does not.

Perhaps you worry that your parent, partner, child, or friend will just fade away in a facility. Consider that the people who work in dementia care communities are prepared to engage with and entertain their residents. There are activities and entertainers designed specifically for people with dementia. Your dad with dementia, for example, will not just sit there, bored, on a couch all day.

Consider, as well, that your dad with dementia does not live in the same world that you do. He exists on another planet, a planet where time is confusing, and his exact relationship with it is mixed up. Those with dementia live in the world they lived in years ago—their children are young, they are working for a living, and they are still married. At a dementia care community, a person with dementia has the opportunity to live in that world. All good care communities have a reason for offering baby dolls, realistic-looking stuffed animals, and other life-skills stations that resemble things we would see out in the real world.

Consider, too, that you, as a caregiver, can have a better life when your family member or friend lives in long-term care. Maybe this feels like a selfish reason to choose a community for someone, but it's a decision that will ensure the best care for yourself and your family member. It is difficult to provide the best possible care when you as a caregiver are stressed and unhappy.

DEMENTIA DOES NOT HAVE TO BE TERRIBLE

Although dementia is distressing, a person who has dementia does not have to lead a terrible existence. People with dementia have the opportunity to live out happy, healthy, and fulfilling lives in care communities. People with dementia live in a different world than we do—a world with the possibility of being a much happier place than the real world. Instead of being 90 years old and riddled with physical ailments, a woman with dementia believes that she is 25 and still in the prime of her life.

"We had a great time today," Alexis told me as we walked down the hallway.

"Oh, yeah?" I asked. "What were you all doing?"

"My group of gals and I went dancing at this senior community," Alexis said, smiling. "The old folks really seemed to enjoy it, too. They were clapping and laughing and dancing. It was really a beautiful moment, wish you coulda been there."

Alexis had dementia and lived in our care community. She had been, at one point in her life, a dancer. From what I gathered, she was really quite the star, too. Alexis had danced all over New York City and Broadway.

This day, in particular, Alexis's mind had convinced her that she had been dancing at a senior-living community. This story was funny because she *had* been dancing at a senior community—her own community, where she lived. Alexis had seen the older faces in the crowd as she cruised across the floor, dancing in time to the beat of the accordion player. She had seen the older adults— her friends, her companions—get up and dance with her. Alexis believed that she and her dancing group had volunteered at a senior-living community, but really, she had just been dancing on her own dementia care floor.

She regularly regaled us with stories of her younger days, even though they were always in the present tense. Alexis believed, without a doubt, that she currently lived that life she had loved so very much. She was still a dancer. She was still a young woman— meeting men, laughing, going out, eating fabulous dinners, and engaging in interesting conversation. She was not an 85-year-old woman who sometimes fell asleep on our activity room couch with no shoes on. Alexis was not a confused woman who needed help showering and organizing her closet. She was not a woman who needed to be escorted to the dining room so she would not forget where it was. Alexis was, in her world, an adventurer living her life to the fullest. And we believed that, too.

Notes

Chapter 3. What Type of Dementia Is It, and Why Does It Matter?

1. Budson, A. E. & Kowall, N. W. (2014). *The Handbook of Alzheimer's Disease and Other Dementias*. West Sussex, UK: John Wiley & Sons, Ltd. (p. 5).
2. Ibid., pp. 4–5.
3. Ibid., p. 198.
4. Ibid., pp. 146–149.
5. Ibid., pp. 146–149.
6. Ibid., pp. 150–151.
7. Ibid., pp. 151–154.
8. Ibid., pp. 92–97.
9. Ibid., p. 131.
10. Ibid., p. 133.
11. Ibid., p. 180.
12. Ibid., p. 34.

Chapter 22. Day Trips and Outings

1. Alzheimer's Association. (2015). *Seven Stages of Alzheimer's*. Retrieved from www.alz.org/alzheimers_disease_stages_of _alzheimers.asp.

Index

accidents, 10, 18, 28, 81, 185

activities in community, 5, 23–24, 26, 27, 72-76; to bring joy, 76–77; engagement in, 4, 24, 25–26, 70, 71–72, 94, 106, 114, 193; lack of, 69–70; on move-in day, 106; to prevent sundowning, 139–40; and search for right community, 70–72

activities of daily living (ADLs), 10, 12, 96, 99

activity director, 30, 71–72, 87, 143, 144

addressing person with dementia, 48–49, 147, 151–52

adult day care centers, 3, 95, 190

aggression, 19, 54, 105, 130–32, 157–63; approach to person exhibiting, 160–63; coping with, 159–60; due to pain, delirium, or illness, 163; sundowning and, 136, 139, 160; triggers for, 160

agitation, 37, 42, 55, 69, 70, 85, 132, 162; aggression and, 157; effect of music on, 88; related to moving in, 106–7; sundowning and, 6, 136–41

Alzheimer's Association, 146

Alzheimer's disease, 8, 9, 11–13, 16, 17, 18, 24, 128; early-onset, 12; family interactions and, 45, 111; friendships and, 117–19, 121; moving someone with, 108; outings for persons with, 142; phrase repetition and, 175; stages of, 12–13; symptoms of, 9, 12, 14, 53

amnestic syndrome, 8

anger: of family, 28, 50, 96, 102, 152, 187; of staff, 43

anger of person with dementia, 13, 36, 61, 75, 132, 158; about being moved, 103, 104, 108; coping with, 159; due to pain/illness, 132, 163; when family leaves, 111, 112

anxiety of family/visitors, 6, 86, 109, 144

anxiety of person with dementia, 43, 45, 54, 58, 63, 70, 77, 79, 81, 104; due to UTI, 55, 132; sundowning and, 6

aphasia, 170, 178. *See also* language/speech problems

assisted-living facilities (ALFs), 3, 4, 23–26, 142, 189

baking/cooking activities, 5, 87, 142

bathing/showering, 10, 12, 21, 93, 100

About the Author

Rachael Wonderlin received her bachelor of science in psychology from the University of Mary Washington. While attending college, Rachael's love and passion for mental health grew as she learned more about the mind. After graduating, Rachael moved to North Carolina and began her master's degree in gerontology, which she earned in 2013, at the University of North Carolina at Greensboro.

She has since worked in hospitals, skilled-nursing facilities, home care, Area Agencies on Aging, and assisted-living communities. Rachael now applies her knowledge and care to residents at a long-term dementia care community. Although she realizes that not everyone shares her passion for dementia care, Rachael wants to inspire others to improve their relationships with adults who have dementia.

To read more about Rachael's experiences in long-term dementia care communities, please visit her blog, Dementia by Day, at *dementia -by-day.com*.